What They're Saying...

"Consumer demand for natural medicine is at an unprecedented level. Herbs represent the fastest growing segment of sales in the mainstream marketplace today.

This handbook provides much-needed information on some of the leading herbs in the market to help pharmacists deal with the exploding consumer demand for information on the responsible use of herbal dietary supplements.

Consumers will also benefit immensely from this book's wealth of valuable, well-researched information!"

Mark Blumenthal, Executive Director,
Editor and Publisher of HerbalGram,
Founder and Executive Director of the
American Botanical Council, Austin, TX

"Two years ago, after having lupus for 20 years, I was diagnosed with breast cancer. Steve came into my life and changed it forever. His herbal therapy enabled me to get through chemotherapy and has built up my immune system. Thanks to Steve, I am living and enjoying life again."

Barbara Simoneau, Londonderry, NH

"After years of allergies, specialists, prescriptions, and headaches, I listened to Steve's advice about herbs. This is my most allergy-free spring in years!"

Abbyann Carr, Henniker, NH

"The use of herbal remedies has become commonplace, and more often than not, patients do not mention their use of herbal remedies to their doctors or pharmacists for fear of ridicule. Clinicians should ask their patients about any herbal (or other types of) therapy in order to better care for them. However most clinicians do not know much about herbal therapy and are therefore reluctant to ask.

Medicinal Herbal Therapy by Steven Ottariano offers clinicians a concise review of herbal therapy which will allow them to counsel and caution their patients who may be using herbal products.

The book is written by a pharmacist in scientific language that is easily understood by clinicians, and unlike many books on herbal and "alternative" therapies available today, is based upon the published medical literature. Mr. Ottariano presents both the good and the bad of herbal therapies without the anecdotal hyperbole that is often found in popular books.

For clinicians who are interested in recommending herbal products for their patients, Medicinal Herbal Therapy will also serve as an excellent guide that can be trusted. Mr. Ottariano has produced an outstanding book that will be of interest to nearly all physicians and pharmacists. It is the best book I have seen on this topic. It should be in all medical libraries, pharmacies and doctors' offices."

Errol Green, M.D., R.Ph., FACEP
Assistant Professor of Emergency Medicine,
Tufts University School of Medicine,
and Assistant Chief of Emergency Medicine,
New England Medical Center, Boston, MA

"Steve is an amazingly competent authority on the subject of the healing powers of herbs. He has given me excellent advice in the use of herbs for various health issues, ranging from menstrual cramps to general health issues. He has made me more aware of the natural alternatives to conventional pharmaceuticals. I have the utmost respect for Steve and his knowledge in this field."

Kathleen Yeager, Londonderry, NH

"Having injured my left knee and failing at traditional treatment prescribed by my doctor, I turned to Steve for help. I took his advice to use natural herbal remedies to treat my knee. After treatment with herbs, my knee has retained 97 percent function.
I was amazed that herbs could help!"

Dana G., Manchester, NH

MEDICINAL

❧ HERBAL

THERAPY ❧

MEDICINAL
❧ HERBAL
THERAPY❧

A Pharmacist's Viewpoint

Steven G. Ottariano, R.Ph.

Foreword by Marc Levenson, M.D.
Illustrations by Joyce Orchard Garamella

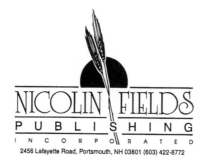

NICOLIN FIELDS
PUBLISHING
INCORPORATED
2456 Lafayette Road, Portsmouth, NH 03801 (603) 422-8772

Notice: This book is designed to educate and as a reference for many of the most common and clinically tested herbs that exist today. It is not a self-diagnostic reference. In no way is it intended to be a substitute for qualified medical intervention, counseling, or testing. Neither the publisher nor the author shall be held liable or responsible to any person or living entity for injury, damage, error, or loss that may be caused (or alleged to be caused) directly or indirectly by the information contained in this book.

Medicinal Herbal Therapy A Pharmacist's Viewpoint. Copyright © 1999 by Steven G. Ottariano, R.Ph. Published by Nicolin Fields Publishing, Inc., 2456 Lafayette Road, Portsmouth, NH 03801. Email address: nfp@nh.ultranet.com.

Illustrations copyright © 1999 by Joyce Orchard Garamella
Author photograph copyright © 1999 Linda Chestney
Cover designer: Joyce Weston
Interior designer: Linda Chestney

First Edition, Second Printing

Library of Congress Cataloging-in-Publication Data

Ottariano, Steven G., 1949-
    Medicinal herbal therapy : a pharmacist's viewpoint / Steven
G. Ottariano ; foreword by Marc Levenson ; illustrations by
Joyce Orchard Garamella. -- 1st ed.
      p.   cm.
    Includes bibliographical references and index.
    ISBN 0-9637077-6-0
    1. Herbs--Therapeutic use. I. Title.
RM666.H33088 1999   98-22339
615' .321--dc21   CIP

To my wife, Anne,
My children, Jason and Stephanie.
And to my second family
at the House of the Samurai
Shidokan International.

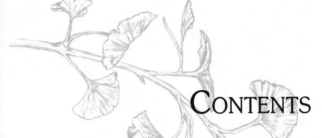

Contents

Part One
What Ails You?

PART TWO
THE HEALING HERBS

PART THREE
TOPICAL HERBAL TREATMENTS

PART FOUR
APPENDIXES

ACKNOWLEDGEMENTS

To the staff at the Veterans Affairs Medical Center (VAMC), Manchester, New Hampshire, especially the Department of Pharmacy, whose encouragement kept this project alive and well.

To doctors Hugh Bower, Madeline Gerken, Keith Jorgensen, Marc Levenson, Alex Montiero, Johann Rothwangl.

To pharmacists Mark Connelly, Tom Bonito, Jeanne Demers and George Kenson.

To nurses Barbara Bernard, Amy Guthrie, Linda Powers, and Gail Vanark.

To Hanshi Ritchie Bernard, Carl and Diane Fitzgerald, Eppy Gray, Bert Lombard, Annie Potter, Chuck Powers, and Guy and Kathy Yeager for their support and comments.

To Mark Blumenthal, Executive Director of the American Botanical Council, and editor of one of the best periodicals on herbal therapy, *HerbalGram*, for his valuable time and guidance.

To Dr. June Riedlinger, Pharm.D., Assistant Professor of Clinical Pharmacy, Massachusetts College of Pharmacy, Boston, MA for her clinical contributions.

To my publisher, Linda Chestney, who started this whole thing by asking, "Did you ever think of writing a book?"

I am always ready to learn, but I do not always like being taught.

~Sir Winston Churchill
(1874-1965)

FOREWORD

Why is it now, after a 100-year revolution in medical science, that Western medicine is becoming more interested in remedies dating back thousands of years? I think there are ` two factors at work. First, the healthcare consumer has become more "activist" and is less likely to accept the paternalism of past medical practice. They demand answers from whatever source.

Second, I believe more and more members of the medical community feel that the therapeutics of Western medical science are incomplete and potentially more toxic than natural remedies. While not totally innocuous, most natural remedies have a much lower incident of side effects, including serious short and long-term side effects, than many manufactured pharmaceuticals. (Having said this, I recall the case of a patient who experienced a dangerously low platelet count from consuming a large amount of chrysanthemum tea—but such examples are extremely rare.) Most consumers are turning to herbal remedies as preventatives and as a complement to manufactured medicine.

In this regard, I applaud Mr. Ottariano's approach, which does not castigate manufactured medicines, but sees the two types of substances enhancing each other. I found reading this book extremely informative. It is well researched.

Lack of investigation as to potency and side effects has always been the most severe criticism of herbal remedies, but I think books like this one, which survey the existing scientific literature, will do much to vitiate this criticism.

I think this book should be a reference for every medical practitioner in this country and deserves a place next to the *Physicians' Desk Reference* in every medical library.

Marc Levenson, M.D., Chief of Staff,
Veterans Affairs Medical Center, Manchester, NH

THE BEGINNING OF MEDICINAL HERBAL THERAPY:

MEDICINAL PLANTS OF OUR MAINE INDIANS

(According to Chief Needahbeh, Librarian of Penobscot Tribe (1934), as told to Lucinda Lombard)

When the first white men came, as wilderness wayfarers, and saw an Indian and his squaw gathering roots and herbs, they did not realize the great preponderance of tradition, prayer formula, and plant myths behind their actions. A fascinating and charming plant lore was and is existent here among them and its origin goes back to the beginning of things. Great storytellers of their race reveal the interesting legends, which have grown up around them.

From Darkness Into the Light

According to them, the animals and birds, plants and trees, all existed before man and were very powerful. At that time men lived underground. The Blue Bird found the place where man came up from the darkness and into the light.

As time went on, because of endless hunting, the animals and birds grew antagonistic toward the man. So they held a council and many resolved to each bring a disease to man to punish him.

But the plants and trees favored him, and sought to intervene offering to those who were wise enough to understand their language, the juice and sap of their leaves and bark to

alleviate suffering. Many animals and birds also availed themselves of this privilege.

The souls of trees and plants told what was good for those
who loved them rightly and each member of the plant-tribe
had a special mission to perform—except a few renegades like
poison ivy. The plants' council house was under the dome of
Mt. Katahdin. The underground world from whence they sprang
was similar to our upper world, except the seasons were different. For is not spring water warm in winter and cold in summer?

Observing Nature at Work

To learn their uses was attained in two ways. The first method
was to watch how animals regulated the interior working of their
bodies. When spring comes, the winged insects fly to the wil-
lows where they use the catkin pollen for internal cleansing. Bears,
after their long winter's sleep, eat mandrake leaves before they
eat food. Indian dogs ate certain herbs for indigestion and others
for intestinal cleansing. A colony of crows knew how to find an
antidote for some poisonous berries their young had eaten—
another species of berries caused them to vomit. A toad bitten
by a spider finds leaves to creep under and wind about him to
remove the poison.

The second method was by prayer and fasting, and by following the crystal trails of the streams back to the hills or down
to the sea, where so many healing herbs grew.

In gathering very valuable and less common plants, such as
mandrake, bloodroot, spotted pipsissewa, the small and large
yellow lady's slipper, etc., the Medicine Man directed that the
first three plants be passed by, but the fourth gathered. Seeds of
these were planted in their habitats "to appease their discour-
aged spirits."

The fir tree possessed a supernatural power of strength. Its
tips were used for rubbing while bathing, cleansing them spiri-
tually and preparing them for prayer. Lodges of its boughs were
made, rocks heated, and cold water poured on them for sweat
treatments for colds, rheumatism and cramps. Hot drinks of fir
tea were given simultaneously.

A ceremony, appealing in its poetic meaning, applies to white clover. Very soon after a child was born, this plant—whose Indian name was "it follows every man's footsteps"—was pulverized and put in crystal-clear water from a noisy waterfall. This was given to the baby for four days for a retentive memory.

These hardy people acclimated to their rock-bound land with its deep snows and mountains and lakes. They knew sickness and accident so well that their whole religion was centered upon one big purpose: *healing*—their biggest need and desire.

Ancient Remedies

Their stone-age creed looked to the Medicine Man with his chants and drums in the darkness of night, his fasts and prayers, and his occult power of medicine, to conquer the powers of evil. Deep-seated in the Indian is the belief that bodily ill is due to getting out of tune with the Great Spirit.

Their Medicine Man was born to be a healer, so he brought back the age of miracles, a part of their faith in the Great Spirit. After all, faith is a most satisfying possession, and our modern medicine is scarcely more logical.

The Indians believed (as did our ancestors) in the "doctrine of signatures," i.e., that the form and color of plants pointed out their uses. For instance, jaundice was treated with a decoction of the barberry, a yellowish-colored plant. The cranesbill (geranium) whose leaves turn red in dying was used to heal wounds. Bloodroot was good for blood diseases. Liverwort healed liver troubles, including coughs, its leaves being three-lobed, as is that organ. The red roots of the black willow are used for blood purifying. Goat's rue (*Galega officinalis*), "devil's thongs" (*Cracca virginiana*), because "its stem was so strong," was made into an ointment for strengthening the muscles of the young braves.

When we realize that 60 percent of our present-day pharmacists' recipes are compounded from Indian remedies, we see the immense amount of valuable Aboriginal knowledge which has been given to civilization.

❧❧❧

*The art of medicine consists of
amusing the patient
while nature cures the disease.*

~Francois-Marie Arouet Voltaire
(1694-1778)

INTRODUCTION:
WHO IS THIS BOOK FOR?

Your first reaction to this book may be, "Oh no, not another book on herbs!" Well yes, but not exactly.

When I began my pharmacist's studies at Northeastern University, all resemblance of any courses that taught pharmacognosy (the study of the medicinal components of plants and their use in medicine), had all but disappeared or had been delegated to the elective status (provided you could find someone to teach it). Synthetic preparations had been developed to treat everything from high-blood pressure to eczema. Any mention of plant derivatives was usually in the context of what was done in the "olden days," which to some meant during the last Ice Age. This was, unfortunately, the way it was taught in medical and pharmacy colleges since right after World War II.

During this time frame of manufactured pharmaceuticals, I was being treated by an allergist for my allergies and asthma. I had developed asthma at 10 years of age and at 12, I went into respiratory arrest and traveled down the big, black tunnel toward the big, bright "Light." (I never really talked about my little trip to the "other side" until Dr. Elizabeth Kubler-Ross published her book, *On Death and Dying*.)

My allergist said that we had tried everything that was out there for medications, and then he mentioned some "other" therapies he'd been reading about—including breathing exercises, herbs, nutritional programs, and acupuncture. He said that he would only mention them because even though they had been tested and used in Europe and Asia, he couldn't suggest their use because they hadn't been given the FDA seal-of-approval. He also mentioned that he didn't want to be known as a "quack" by the rest of the medical community for putting his patients on these therapies. Medical students were never taught about these therapies in school, he said. If I wanted to look into them, I was pretty much on my own. I asked how he knew of these "alternatives" and other physicians didn't. His response was that he was introduced to these "different" therapies while visiting Europe and Asia. (Fortunately, today more medical, pharmacy and nursing colleges are teaching alternative medicine than they did 50 years ago.)

On My Own...

So I decided to look into some of these therapies. I was curious to see if any of them really worked or were just "old wives' tales." Well I must say, the "old wives" knew what they were talking about.

My asthma is gone and I am not on any medication. It was one of several types of therapies I used. I learned to breathe from the diaphragm through Martial Arts training. I adjusted my diet. I used herbs when I had an acute asthmatic attack—along with my inhalers. I found that by combining prescription medications with these new (old) therapies, I got the best of both worlds. I was able to take control of the asthma and not allow it to control me.

As you can see, I made the choice to try these alternative therapies on my own. Until recently, this was how most people chose these types of remedies. Their family physician would never mention it to them because 1) he/she didn't know about them, and 2) they probably had no scientific basis for use. The patient always sought out the therapies themselves. Insurance companies wouldn't pay for any of these services (although many do now) so the patient had to pay for them from his/her own pocket.

It seems strange to me that the United States, one of the most technologically advanced nations in the world, also has the highest medical percentage of Gross National Product in the world. What are we doing wrong?

Complementary Therapies

Well luckily these "complementary therapies" have come out into the light. (I like the use of the term "complementary" instead of "alternative.") All medical options should complement one another and be used with the ultimate goal of helping the patient. We are now learning what was known in the past, and with today's technology, we are able to confirm many of these findings.

This book will deal with one complementary therapy—herbs. What I have attempted to do in this book is eliminate what I call the "Grandma Factor." Grandma may have used an herb for her family many years ago and it may have worked. But there may not have been any clinical studies conducted on that herb. That doesn't necessarily mean that it is unsafe. It just means that in today's society we need a little more evidence before we can safely recommend its use. There are many herbs that we still need to look at more carefully.

I've chosen to focus on the herbs that I have used in my counseling practice with which I've had great success. Additionally I have supported the suggestions with documented scientific studies in reference sections throughout the book. I have also specifically limited this work to Western herbalism. I will not be discussing Chinese herbalism and its vast use of formulas nor will I be going into the use of nutritional or homeopathic medicine.

Which Form is Best?

Within the world of herbalism you will find many that differ as to which form of an herb is best. Should it be in tea? A capsule? A tablet, liquid, tincture, or…? From a pharmacist's viewpoint, the magic word is "compliance." You may have a cure for every disease known to humankind but if the tablet or capsule is too big or the elixir gives you an upset stomach just from the smell, you will never take it.

Take the form that is the most comfortable for you. If you can't swallow tablets, take the tincture. If the tincture is inconvenient, try the capsules (some exceptions are mentioned in the book). It doesn't matter what form it's in, *just as long as it is taken!* Noncompliance is one of the biggest problems—even with prescription drugs. Medications won't work unless they are physically inside your body.

Are They Safe?

This brings me to another viewpoint. Don't be fooled into thinking that just because these "medicinals" come from plants they must be safer than prescription drugs and you can take more. This concept couldn't be further from the truth. Any medicinal herb that you take alters the chemical reaction that occurs inside your body.

Some herbs can interfere with or add to the effects of other medications (e.g., valerian and alprazolam), or could worsen an already existing condition (e.g., ma huang and high-blood pressure). Even though I've included such information with each herb, one should always ask a qualified clinician if any of these herbs will interfere with one's current regimen of prescription medications, over-the-counter preparations (OTCs), and other herbs.

Standardization

This is probably the most important item that can be discussed from a clinician's standpoint. If you purchase an herb from one company and then purchase the same herb from another company, you would think that the ingredients would be consistent. Unfortunately, this is not necessarily true. Herbal potency can vary greatly.

Herbs are not strictly regulated the way prescription drugs are, although many herbal companies have as strict as, or better, standards. For this reason you should look for products which state that they have a standardized potency on the label. With today's technology, science can analyze the different compounds in the plant. Therefore we should know within what range of potency they should be in order to achieve the desired effects. I don't want to see us extracting one particular ingredient and using only that one. Herbs work best when all the other compounds are used in synergy with one another. But we need to have a foundation in order to start.

The Healing Herbs

So, if you are looking for a book to teach you how to make teas, fill capsules, make liniments, creams or a poultice, then you would be wise to look elsewhere. There are many excellent books on these subjects listed in the resource section. But if you want to take charge of your health care, then read on. If you want to know about some of the most widely used and clinically significant herbs, how they work and how to use them, then this book will well serve your needs.

In closing, it would be wise for everyone, whether clinicians or laity, to absorb the knowledge of how the herbal kingdom can help humankind. The answers are right in front of our eyes and have already been put on this earth. It's our job to find and apply them properly.

Steve Ottariano, R.Ph.

PART ONE

WHAT
AILS YOU?

WHAT AILS YOU?

There is an old saying that states that if you take antibiotics for two weeks your cold will go away. If you take nothing, the cold will go away in 14 days!

Our bodies contain miraculous powers to heal themselves. And it seems that the more natural the source (and in most cases you don't need the strongest)—the faster the body heals—and with fewer side effects.

In this section, you will find herbal therapies to use for particular problems.

Additionally, check under the *The Healing Herbs* Section (Part Two) for more information on herbs that are mentioned in *this* section.

Acne

Y ou don't have to be a teenager to have an "acne attack."
Those unsightly blemishes can come at any age and on
any part of the body.

Sebaceous glands secrete oil, which helps to lubricate the skin.
When they become clogged, bacteria can begin to grow and
cause the skin to erupt. No definite cause is known, but diet,
hygiene, and hormones may play a role in its development.

Use:

• **Tea Tree Oil** (externally)—Apply to affected area 2 to 3 times
a day

For additional information on tea tree oil, check the Topical
Herbal Treatments (Part Three) section of this book.

Allergies

A n allergic reaction develops when the body's normal defense mechanism overreacts. A substance that would not
normally cause a problem is treated by the immune system as
an "enemy" that must be destroyed. The body therefore mus-
ters up its army of white blood cells to attack the intruder. But
this hyperactivity causes more harm than good.

The allergic reaction can manifest itself externally (e.g., a rash),
or internally, as asthma. The intruder is known as an "aller-
gen." Allergens can be anything from dust to pollen or numerous other irritants as well. When the white blood cells break
open, they release substances that cause the allergic reactions.

Many herbs help prevent the cell walls from breaking down and releasing these substances into the blood stream.

Use:

- **Evening Primrose Oil** (EPO) —500mg to 1000mg 3 to 4 times a day
- **Garlic**—3000mcg (micrograms of allicin content) daily
- **Ginkgo Biloba**—40mg to 80mg 3 times a day
- **Quercetin**—500mg 2 to 4 times a day
- **Stinging Nettle Root**—250mg to 500mg 3 to 4 times a day

Anxiety

Anxiety has unfortunately become synonymous with our modern society. Not that other generations didn't have their times of stress and tension, it just seems that we are more aware of the mental and physical problems which can occur from unresolved stress.

We all experience stress. The difference is in how we handle it. All of us have "stressors"—little things that can build up and cause our bodies to react in physical ways—such as an increase in blood pressure which could lead to cardiac and circulatory problems, intestinal disorders like gas and diarrhea, as well as headaches and muscle spasms, just to name a few.

Herbs such as chamomile, kava, St. John's wort and valerian can help balance the equation of our daily lives.

Use:

- **Chamomile**—350mg to 500mg in capsule form 3 to 4 times a day. If desired, a tea can be made by breaking the capsules open and dissolving the contents in hot water.
- **Kava**—100mg 2 to 3 times a day

- **St. John's Wort**—300mg 2 to 3 times a day
- **Valerian**—150mg to 300mg 2 to 3 times a day

Arthritis

M any herbal products have shown promise in helping to relieve the pain and swelling of both osteoarthritis and rheumatoid arthritis.

Osteoarthritis is the deterioration of the cartilage in between the joints due to age, wear, and tear.

Rheumatoid arthritis can affect any age group. The cartilage and synovial fluid in between the joints breaks down and causes the bones to fuse and become swollen and disfigured. Often you can see its deformity in the joints along the fingers. The knees are another area that can become affected which can make everyday tasks, such as walking and standing, extremely painful.

Although considered more as nutrients rather than herbs, glucosamine sulphate (500 mg 3 times daily) and chondroitin sulphate (400 mg 3 times daily) have shown results in helping to strengthen what cartilage is left between the joints.

Use:
- **Bromelain**—500mg (between meals) 3 times a day
- **Capsaicin Cream**—Apply externally up to 5 times a day
- **Feverfew**—400 mcg to 800mcg of a standardized form 3 times a day
- **Ginger**—500mg to 1000mg 3 to 4 times a day
- **Quercetin**—500mg 3 to 4 times a day

Asthma

(See also Respiratory Tract Disorders)

The latest definition from the 1995 National Heart, Lung and Blood/World Health Organization Workshop report states that asthma is "a chronic inflammatory disorder of the airways."

This can include airway hyper-responsiveness due to an allergy, infection, or it can be exercise-induced. Airflow limitations and respiratory symptoms such as wheezing, coughing and tightness in the chest can develop when the muscles around the lungs constrict and the air flow becomes harder to enter and leave the body. The lungs need the muscles around them and below them—the diaphragm—in order to work.

When asthma is caused by allergies, mast cells release histamine and other chemicals into the blood stream to cause further constriction. (A mast cell is a cell, which when it feels attacked, releases histamine, an inflammatory compound.)

Many herbs have been shown to relax the bronchial muscle spasms and prevent the mast cells from breaking down.

Use:

- **Deglycyrrhizinated licorice (DGL)** —helps to increase the function of the adrenals—take 250mg to 500mg 3 to 4 times a day

- **Evening Primrose Oil**—helpful in the treatment of eczema
    - Children—250mg to 500mg 3 times a day
    - Adults—500mg to 1000mg 3 to 4 times a day

- **Garlic**—3000mcg to 5000mcg (micrograms of allicin content) daily

- **Ginkgo Biloba**—helps to prevent the release of platelet-activating factor (PAF) which may cause broncho-constriction. Consider taking 40mg to 80mg 3 times a day

- **Lobelia and Ma Huang**—Follow the manufacturer's directions **EXACTLY.** Use under the guidance of a trained clinician.
- **Quercetin**—500mg 3 to 4 times a day
- **Stinging Nettle Root**—250mg 3 times a day

Asthma: Take it Seriously

The above-mentioned herbs may be used with standard medications to help in the treatment of asthma. Asthma is a very serious illness, and unfortunately, can be fatal. It should never be considered as a "do-it-yourself home improvement project" that can be treated with herbs alone.

In some cases a person may be allergic to an herb and could therefore make the situation worse. Asthma should be approached from a multi-pointed attack. Diet (eliminate milk and cheese), breathing exercises, regular physical exercise (swimming and the Martial Arts are especially beneficial), relaxation techniques, proper use of inhalers and spacers, and the use of peak-flow meters, are just a few of the methods that can be used to help control the symptoms of asthma.

Other herbs and therapies that may be of benefit include:

- **Acupuncture**
- **Echinacea, Astragalus, and Garlic**—help to boost the immune system to guard against developing respiratory infections.
- **Magnesium**—although this is not an herb, studies have shown that asthmatics have very low blood levels of this important mineral. Adults—250mg to 750mg daily A good rule of thumb is to have the magnesium equal half the amount of calcium.
- **Shiatsu** (Japanese acupressure)

By combining many of these therapies, the control of asthma can be in your hands.

Atherosclerosis

Atherosclerosis is the narrowing of the arteries due to the formation of fatty plaque that develop deposits (mostly from our diet). This constricts the flow of blood to the rest of the body and makes the heart work harder.

This can lead to all sorts of problems such as high-blood pressure, angina, and myocardial infarction (MI). An MI is a full-blown heart attack whereby the vessels become completely blocked either by these fatty deposits or a blood clot. Along with diet and exercise, there are certain herbs that can help decrease the risk of blood vessels constricting.

Use:

* **Dandelion**—500mg to 1000mg 3 to 4 times a day
* **Garlic**—3000mcg (micrograms of allicin content) daily
* **Ginger**—500mg to 1000mg 3 to 4 times a day
* **Ginkgo Biloba**—40mg to 80mg 3 times a day
* **Gugulipid**—25mg 3 times a day
* **Hawthorn**—Start with 80mg twice daily (May increase slowly as needed to 160mg 3 times a day)

Benign Prostatic Hyperplasia (BPH)

Benign prostatic hyperplasia is a serious, though not cancerous, disorder. It develops when the prostate becomes enlarged and therefore constricts the natural flow of urine through the urethra.

34

This constriction of urine can also back up through the ureters to the kidneys and can cause infection such as cystitis. Herbal and nutrient therapy can help with this condition.

Use:

- **Saw Palmetto**—160mg 2 times a day
- **Stinging Nettle Root**—250mg to 500mg 3 times a day
- **Zinc**—50mg to 100mg daily

Candidiasis

*C*andida albicans is a yeast-like fungus that normally inhabits the mucous membranes of the body (for example the intestines, genito-urinary and respiratory). It usually poses no problem unless it is allowed to grow out of proportion to the rest of the healthy flora that inhabit our bodies. This can happen by taking antibiotics whose job it is to kill bacteria. Unfortunately antibiotics do not know the difference between the good bacteria (*Lactobacillus acidophilus*) and the bad bacteria that is causing the infection. It just kills all susceptible bacteria and therefore allows *Candida albicans* to take over the environment of the mucous membranes.

Other factors that favor its growth are a diet high in refined sugars (which weaken the immune system), birth-control pills, and steroids. Outbreaks of candidiasis usually can be seen as white pockets in the mouth (thrush) and as a white discharge from the vagina. But it can also manifest itself with symptoms of fatigue, headache, diarrhea, gas, constipation and allergies, just to name a few.

Use:

- **Echinacea**—30 drops of a standardized tincture or 300mg to 600mg 3 times a day

- **Garlic**—3000mcg to 5000mcg (micrograms of allicin content) daily
- **Goldenseal**—250mg to 500mg 3 to 4 times a day

Canker Sores

Canker sores are small painful ulcers (apthous ulcers) that occur inside the mouth. They can form on the inside of the cheeks, lips and gums, and can last from anywhere seven to 21 days. The painful sores are usually brought on by a deficient immune system, allergies, stress, or fatigue. Cold sores or fever blisters are caused by the Herpes simplex virus (Type 1) and can be highly contagious. The treatment for an oral outbreak is the same as for canker sores.

Use:

- **Deglycyrrhizinated Licorice** (DGL) **lozenges**—250mg to 500mg 3 times a day
- **Chamomile and Echinacea** as a mouthwash—Rinse mouth 2 to 3 times a day

Cataracts

Cataracts form when the normally clear lens of the eye becomes cloudy and results in distorted vision in both near and distant objects. This is due to free-radical damage.

The majority of cataracts are seen in the over-60-year-old population, but can also be caused by steroids, diabetes, and overexposure to the sun's ultraviolet rays. In some cases, surgery may be needed in order to correct the vision.

Use:

• **Bilberry**—80mg to 160mg 3 times a day

Cerebrovascular Disorders

I nsufficient blood flow to the brain reduces the amount of oxygen it receives. This can lead to all sorts of problems—especially for the elderly.

Lack of oxygen to the brain can manifest itself with symptoms of fatigue, disorientation, loss of memory, depression, and confusion.

Many of these symptoms may be lumped together and diagnosed (or misdiagnosed), as Alzheimer's disease.

Use:

• **Ginkgo Biloba**—40mg to 80mg 3 times a day

Constipation

T ake a walk down any health and beauty-aid aisle and you would be amazed at how Madison Avenue has tried to convince us that the best seat in the house is still in the bathroom.

Our obsession with "potty priority" has developed into a multi-million-dollar industry. Mother Nature may at times need a little help, but most cases of constipation fall under preventive medicine.

Constipation results when the solid waste (feces) moves too slowly through the intestines. This results in infrequent and difficult bowel movements. The longer the feces stays in the colon, the more water is absorbed by the body from the stool, and this makes it harder to eliminate. This also forces the person to strain which could cause hemorrhoids, and can even raise the blood pressure, which could cause serious consequences.

Fecal toxins can also be absorbed back into the bloodstream. The normal transit time for food entering the body is between 18 and 24 hours.

It is surprising how just a change in diet (more fiber and less refined foods), exercise, and an increase in fluid may solve most of the "constipation blues." Herbal laxatives are primarily bulk-forming laxatives or stimulant laxatives.

Bulk-forming Laxatives

Psyllium seed, also known as plantago seed and plantain, is a frequent component of many bulk-forming, over-the-counter laxatives (e.g., Metamucil®). The seed coats or husks of the plantago seeds contain cells that are filled with mucilage that is neither absorbed nor digested in the intestinal tract. In contact with water it swells to a large volume, thus providing both bulk and lubrication, causing either the whole seed or husks to act as an effective bulk-producing laxative. Obviously, it is necessary to drink large amounts of water when taking this herb.[1,2]

Psyllium comes in both powder and capsule form. If the powder is used, it should be drunk as soon as it is mixed. This will prevent the mixture from thickening before it is swallowed. It may take a few days to see results. Recent studies have also shown that psyllium-enriched cereals may lower total blood-cholesterol readings.[3,4]

Bulk-forming laxatives may also be of some help in the treatment of diarrhea caused by enteral feedings,[5] and in diarrhea caused by irritable bowel syndrome (IBS).

Stimulant Laxatives

Cascara sagrada (*Rhamnus purshiana*), also known as sacred bark, is native to the Pacific Coast of North America. The dried bark of the tree is used medicinally. Cascara's stimulatory action is due to the presence of anthraquinones consisting of cascarosides A, B, C and D. These glycosides increase the peristalsis (muscle contractions) of the intestines. Cascara sagrada is probably the mildest of a class of laxatives called anthraquinones.[6]

Senna (*Cassia angustifolia and Cassia senna*) (e.g., Senokot®) is another stimulant-type, anthraquinone-containing laxative of which the dried fruits and leaves are used for their medicinal properties.

Senna produces a much stronger action than cascara sagrada and therefore can produce increased muscle contractions and intestinal cramping. A senna-fiber combination which equaled two teaspoonfuls (10 ml) daily, was compared to a tablespoonful (15ml) twice daily of the synthetic laxative Lactulose. Improvements in stool frequency, consistency and ease in bowel movement all improved with the use of the senna-combination. It also proved to be more cost-effective.[7]

Dosage and Recommendations:

The dosage for both bulk-forming and stimulant laxatives is based on the specific product used. Often products may contain a combination of ingredients, so the manufacturer's dosage recommendations should be followed. It cannot be overstated enough, however, that these products work best when taken with increased amounts of fluids. A bulk-forming laxative will do just as it should—it will form a massive bulk that will be even harder for the intestines to pass if there is no fluid to help it along.

When we mention exercise to help control constipation, we do not mean that you should go out and run the Boston Marathon. Even in moderation, exercise is effective. For example, in many nursing homes, the gentle Chinese art of Tai Chi is performed with the residents in order to keep them physically active. This not only improves their bowel functions, but also increases their flexibility and improves their outlook on life.

Use:

- **Cascara Sagrada**—Take as recommended on the product that is purchased
- **Psyllium**—Take as recommended on the product that is purchased
- **Senna**—Take as recommended on the product that is purchased

Many herbs may produce a laxative effect. (See Appendix B for additional herbs.)

Herbal Laxatives During Pregnancy

Cautions: Laxatives should only be used under the supervision of a clinician. Nursing mothers should use caution with cascara sagrada and other stimulant laxatives since it does pass through to the mothers' milk and may produce diarrhea in the nursing child.

Psyllium has been reported to interfere with the absorption of the drugs carbamazepine and lithium. It is therefore advisable to take any bulk-forming laxatives at least two hours before or after taking any other medications, herbs, or vitamins.

Internal preparations of aloe have also been used as laxatives. It can produce an extremely strong reaction and should be used with caution. This preparation is not to be confused with the *external* preparations of aloe vera gel.

REFERENCES: CONSTIPATION

1.) Tyler, Varro E
   Herbs of Choice: The Therapeutic Use of Phytomedicinals, pg. 47
   Pharmaceutical Products Press, Binghamton, New York 13904-1580
   © 1994

2.) Tyler VE, Brady LR and Robbers JE
Pharmacognosy, 9th ed.
Lea and Febiger, Philadelphia, 1988 pp. 52-53

3.) Olson BH, Anderson SM, Becker MP, Anderson JW, Hunninghake DB, Jenkins DJA, LaRosa JC, Rippe JM, Roberts DCK, Stoy DB, Summerbell CD, Truswell AS, Wolever TMS, Morris DH, Fulgoni VL Psyllium-Enriched Cereals Lower Blood Total Cholesterol and LDL Cholesterol, but not HDL Cholesterol, in Hypercholesterolemic Adults: Results of a Meta-Analysis
J Nutr 1997 Oct 1; 127 (10): 1973-1980

4.) Belknap D, Davidson LJ, Smith CR
The effects of psyllium hydrophilic mucilloid on diarrhea in enteral fed patients
Heart Lung 1997 May: 26 (3): 229-237

5.) Jenkins DJ, Wolever TM, et al
Effect of psyllium in hypercholesterolemia at two monosaturated fatty acid intakes
Am J Clin Nutr May; 65 (5): 1524-1533, 1997

6.) Tyler, Varro E
Herbs of Choice: The Therapeutic Use of Phytomedicinals, Pg. 48, Pharmaceutical Products Press, Binghamton, New York 13904-1580
© 1994

7.) Passmore AP, Wilson-Davie K, et al
Chronic constipation in long stay elderly patients: a comparison of lactulose and a senna-fiber combination
British Med Journal 307: pp 769-771, 1993

Depression

The word "depression" can describe a vast array of negative signs and symptoms both mental and physical. We all come down with a case of the "blues" once in a while, but it depends on how well we handle it and change it into a brighter color.

Our moods change. We may feel sad, angry and fatigued and may act recklessly all at the same time! Stress can have the same effect. When the stress becomes too much, or more stressors are added, then depression may set in.

Depression is also caused by many *physical* illnesses. Chronic pain or a terminal disease can bring on many psychological and physical changes. It is beyond the scope of this definition to describe all the complications that accompany depression, but if mood and physical changes persist for months instead of weeks, please seek professional therapy.

Use:

- **Ginkgo Biloba**—40mg to 80mg 3 times a day
- **St. John's Wort**—300mg 3 times a day

Diabetes

There are two types of diabetes described in medicine: *diabetes insipidus* and *diabetes mellitis*. *Diabetes insipidus* is a rare disorder caused by a deficiency of the anti-diuretic hormone (ADH) that is produced by the pituitary gland. ADH stimulates the kidneys to reabsorb water.

If the pituitary is damaged by either trauma or illness, not enough ADH is produced and therefore the kidneys will lose water in the form of large amounts of urine. Herbs cannot help with this type of diabetes.

The second and more common diabetes is *diabetes mellitis*. This develops when the pancreas cannot produce sufficient amounts of insulin and therefore the body cannot utilize the glucose in the blood for energy. *Diabetes mellitus* is further divided into Type 1 and Type 2.

Type 1, also called insulin-dependent or juvenile diabetes, usually develops in younger people. Daily insulin shots are given to control the glucose. (Since insulin is a protein molecule, it must be injected. If it were given by mouth, the stomach would digest it as just another protein).

Type 2 is non-insulin-dependent diabetes, or Maturity-Onset Diabetes, is usually seen in middle-aged and older population. This type can usually be controlled by diet, exercise and oral medication, although insulin is sometimes used if all else fails.

Use:

- **Bilberry**—80mg to 160mg 3 times a day
- **Fenugreek**—500mg 4 to 5 times a day
- **Garlic**—2000mcg to 4000mcg (micrograms of allicin content) daily
- **Ginkgo Biloba**—40mg to 80mg 3 times a day
- **Ginseng**—100mg to 500mg 3 times a day
- **Gymnema Sylvestre**—200mg 3 times a day

Diabetes mellitus is usually treated with diet, exercise, oral medication, insulin, or any combination thereof. The following herbs have been shown to help lower the glucose level of the blood. Remember diabetes is not a self-treatable condition. These herbs are a small part of the total treatment picture:

- **Gymnema Sylvestre** *(Meshashringi)*. This herb has been used for many centuries by Ayurvedic practitioners to help reduce blood sugar levels by stimulating the pancreas to produce more insulin.[1,2] In one study, gymnema has shown promise by helping to reduce the need for oral hypoglycemic agents (non-insulin dependent diabetics—Type 2)[1] and it also decreased the amount of insulin used by almost 50 percent in another study[2] (insulin-dependent diabetics—Type 1). The dosage used for both studies was 400 mg daily. This is not a fast-acting herb. It may take a few months to see the benefits.

- **Fennugreek** *(trigonella foenum-graecum)*: The seeds of this herb have been used in both Western herbalism and in Chinese Medicine for healing and have also been used as a spice and a flavoring agent. They contain many compounds which work synergistically to lower blood sugar levels[3] by increasing the ability of erythrocytes to bind insulin.[4] With a dose of 2.5 grams twice daily for three months, fenugreek reduced significantly the blood sugar (fasting and post-prandial) of non-insulin dependent diabetics (Type 2).[5]

Caution:

Fenugreek has been shown to cause an allergic reaction in some people, especially those who are sensitive to any member of the Leguminosae family, which includes chickpeas.[6]

• **Ginkgo Biloba, Bilberry, Garlic and Ginseng.** Ginkgo biloba and bilberry may be used to treat the complications that occur with continued high-blood sugar levels. Both herbs have been shown to help with diabetic retinopathy and diabetic neuropathy. Garlic and ginseng can also be used to help lower blood-sugar levels. (See sections under individual herbs.)

REFERENCES: DIABETES

1.) Baskaran K, et al
Anti-diabetic effect of a leaf extract from Gymnema sylvestre in non-insulin dependent diabetes mellitus patients
J Ethnopharmacol 30: 295-305, 1990

2.) Shanmugasundaram ERB, et al
Use of Gymnema sylvestre leaf extracts in the control of blood glucose in insulin dependent diabetes mellitus
J Ethnopharmacol 30: 281-294, 1990

3.) Ali L, Azad Khan AK, Hassan Z, Mosihuzzaman M, Nahar N, Nasreen T, Nur-e-Alam M, Rokeya B
Characterization of the hypoglycemic effects of Trigonella foenumgraecum seed
Planta Med 1995 Aug; 61 (4): 358-360

4.) Raghuram TC, et al
Effect of fenugreek seeds on intravenous glucose disposition in non-insulin dependent diabetic patients
Phytotherapy Res. 8: 83-86, 1994

5.) Bordia A, Verma SK, Srivastava KC
Effect of ginger (Zingiber officinale Rosc.) and fenugreek (Trigonella foenum-graecum L.) on blood lipids, blood sugar and platelet aggregation in patients with coronary-artery disease
Prostaglandins Leukot Essent Fatty Acids 1997 May; (5): 379-384

6.) Patil SP, Niphadkar PV, Bapat NM
Allergy to fenugreek (Trigonella foenum graecum)
Ann Allergy Asthma Immunol 1997 Mar; 78 (3): 297-300

Diarrhea

D iarrhea develops when the large intestine fails to reabsorb water from the feces. This produces frequency and loose stools. Diarrhea can be caused by many things including foods, parasites, drugs (especially certain antibiotics such as ampicillin), antacids that contain high amounts of magnesium, viruses, and bacteria.

Dehydration is the largest problem associated with diarrhea. Drink plenty of fluids to replace all the vital electrolytes such as potassium. Try not to take medications that will stop the diarrhea, as this is the body's natural defense mechanism to fix the problem unless the diarrhea persists for more than 24 to 36 hours. If diarrhea persists for 48 hours or there is blood in the feces, seek medical help immediately.

Use:
• **Goldenseal**—250mg to 500mg 4 times a day

Eczema

E czema is a superficial skin inflammation characterized by itching, redness, scaling, and sometimes bleeding, if scratched. The word "eczema" is occasionally used synonymously with dermatitis.

Eczema can be of two types: contact or atopic. Contact eczema is caused by an allergic reaction to something that has come in contact with the skin. This can be anything from plants to animals to detergents. Atopic eczema is also caused by allergens but is usually of a chronic nature.

Use:

- **Chamomile**—(externally) Apply to area 3 times a day
- **Ginkgo Biloba**—40mg to 80mg 3 times a day
- **Licorice** (externally)—Apply to area 3 to 4 times a day
- **Quercetin**—500mg to 1000mg 3 to 4 times a day
- **Stinging Nettle Root**—250mg to 500mg 3 to 4 times a day
- **Witch Hazel** (externally)—Apply to area 3 to 4 times a day

Gall Bladder Disorders

The gall bladder can best be described as a "holding" organ. It holds bile from the liver and sends it into the small intestine in response to food. The bile helps with the digestion of fats. It emulsifies, or breaks down, the fat molecules into smaller particles for better utilization for the body.

Use:
- **Dandelion**—500mg to 1000mg 3 to 4 times a day
- **Milk Thistle**—200mg 3 times a day

Gout

Gout is a form of arthritis that develops from an excess of uric acid in the blood stream. The uric acid crystallizes in the joints causing pain and swelling. Most gout sufferers are male.

Diet plays an important role in the treatment. The elimination of purine-containing foods such as red meat, poultry and rich foods, will help control the symptoms. Alcohol also increases the production of uric acid into the blood stream, and so it should be avoided. One must be sure to drink plenty of distilled water—at least one to two liters (a half gallon) daily.

Use:

- **Hawthorn**—80mg to 160mg 3 times a day
- **Stinging Nettle Root**—250mg to 500mg 3 times a day

Gynecological Disorders

(*Also see* the listing under Menopause)

If you are female and have your ovaries intact, then menopause can probably be added to the list of certainties in life, like death and taxes.

As with most things, lack of knowledge and mistruth will always breed fear and contempt. Menopause should not be approached with fear. It is a natural chapter in the book of life. As I stated in the introduction of the book, my philosophy is to try natural options first. If these do not work, you may need a little help from other stronger therapies. This is nowhere more evident than in the case of menopause.

The following herbs have been used in the treatment of menopause and other gynecological disorders:

Helpful Herbs:

• Dong Quai

Dong Quai is the Chinese species of *Angelica*. There are five species of *Angelica*, but only two possess any activity useful for gynecological purposes. They are:

- **Chinese** (Dong Quai) - *Angelica sinensis*

- **Japanese** - *Angelica acutiloba*

The roots and leaves are used medicinally.

Mechanism of Action:

Both the Chinese (*sinensis*) and the Japanese (*acutiloba*) species of *Angelica* contain phytoestrogen compounds. Phytoestrogens compete with estrogen for receptor sites. When estrogen levels are low, they are able to exert some estrogenic activity. When estrogen levels are high, they reduce overall estrogenic activity by occupying estrogen receptor sites.[1] The strength of these phytoestrogens is only 1:400 as active[1] as human estrogen, yet they do exert a considerable effect and may be much safer to use.

Uses:

Dong Quai can be used for the following conditions:

- Dysmenorrhea
- Menopausal symptoms

Dosage:

Take 500mg to 1000mg 2 times daily

Caution:

Since ligustilide is an essential oil found in the herb, which decreases contraction of the smooth muscle of the uterus,[2] Dong Quai should *not* be used during pregnancy. This herb also may produce some photosensitivity.

• Black Cohosh

Black cohosh (*Cimicifuga racemosa*) is a Native American plant and can be found in the Northern Hemisphere. It has also been known as black snakeroot, bugbane (insects seem to be repelled by its odor), squawroot, rattleroot, and rattleweed. Native Americans used it for "female complaints."[3] The roots are used medicinally.

Mechanism of Action:

Black cohosh acts as a phytoestrogen. A clinical study by

Lehmann-Willenbrock and Riedel showed no significant differences among two groups of hysterectomized patients with climacteric symptoms where one group was treated with estrogens and the other with black cohosh.[4]

An alcoholic extract has also been shown to reduce lutenizing hormone (LH) and thus reduce the incidence of hot flashes in menopausal women. The plant has also been shown to have a calming effect and therefore may reduce irritability during times of PMS and menopause.[5,6]

Uses:
Black cohosh may be used to help treat the following conditions:

- Dysmenorrhea
- Menopause (especially hot flashes)
- Premenstrual Syndrome

Dosage:
Take 20mg to 60mg of the standardized extract 3 times daily

Cautions:
Black cohosh may produce some gastrointestinal problems if taken in high doses.

Black cohosh should *not* be used during pregnancy.

Black cohosh (*Cimicifuga racemosa*) should not be confused with blue cohosh (*Caulophylum thalictroides*), which is of a different species. Blue cohosh is reportedly used for many of the same gynecological problems as black cohosh, but has not had as much clinical testing to substantiate its claims.

• Vitex Angus-Castus

Vitex agnus-castus, also known as chaste berry or chaste tree is from the family *Verbenaceae*. The dark, ripe berries are the part of the plant that is used medicinally.

Mechanism of Action:
Vitex agnus-castus increases luteinizing hormone (LH) and mildly inhibits the release of follicle-stimulating hormone (FSH).[7]

Follicle-stimulating hormone and luteinizing hormone are both released from the pituitary gland. LH is responsible for an increase in progesterone levels.

The cause of many premenstrual, menstrual, and menopausal problems may be caused by an imbalance between the amounts of estrogen and progesterone with the shift being in favor of more estrogen and not enough progesterone especially during the luteal phase of the menstrual cycle.

Vitex, therefore, by indirect hormonal action, has the ability to raise progesterone levels and exert a strong corpus-luteum effect.[8] This is in contrast to other phytomedicines, like black cohosh, which bind directly to estrogen receptor sites.[9] Vitex also exerts a lowering of prolactin levels by binding to dopamine receptors and thus inhibit prolactin production by the pituitary.

Uses:

Vitex agnus-castus may be used as primary or complementary therapy in the following disorders:

Menstrual Abnormalities:

- Irregular menstruation (especially if accompanied by endometriosis).[10] This can include:
- Amenorrhea
- Dysmenorrhea
- Hypermenorrhea
- PMS

Premenstrual syndrome can produce a myriad of physical and psychological symptoms. Vitex has been shown to help reduce the effects of depression, mood swings, headache, fatigue, cravings for sweets, breast tenderness, fluid retention and anxiety. Vitex has been shown to work best if these symptoms manifest themselves before menstruation and have a tendency to subside as menstruation progresses.

Other Uses:

Vitex has been shown to decrease the growth of fibroid cysts that occur on smooth muscle tissue or subserous areas. Submucosal cysts *do not* respond to this treatment. Vitex has also been shown to help stabilize the menstrual cycle after withdrawal of birth-control pills containing progesterone.

Because of its effect on prolactin excretion, Vitex has also been used to stimulate lactation in nursing mothers. It seems to work best if taken for the first 10 days after birth.[10,11]

Dosage:

A standardized extract by the name of "agnolyt" has been used in Europe for many years. Forty drops mixed with an ounce of fluid may be given once daily in the morning on an empty stomach. A solid encapsulated extract is also available which contains 175 mg. This also may be taken once daily. Vitex is not fast acting. It is strongly recommended that therapy continue for at least six months for full benefits to be observed.

Cautions:

Vitex should not be used during pregnancy, but can be used to increase lactation. It should not be used for young children. It has no known interactions with other drugs.

• Evening Primrose Oil

Evening Primrose Oil (EPO) (*oenother biennis*) is oil extracted from the seed of the plant. The focus of modern use concentrates on its ability to help with conditions which are associated with prostaglandin deficiencies and metabolism.

Mechanism of Action:

Evening primrose oil is high in gamma linolenic acid (GLA),[12] an essential fatty acid (EFA). Essential fatty acids can only be obtained through our diet. We cannot manufacture them.[13] In our bodies, EFAs undergo a series of complex reactions that convert the EFAs to substances, which can be utilized by the body. Some people have problems with parts of this reaction, especially if they have difficulty utilizing the enzyme delta-6-desaturase. Delta-6-desaturase helps start the beginning part of the reactions that transform EFAs to a form which can be utilized by our bodies[14] so they may be more easily converted to prostaglandins. Prostaglandins help regulate many of the metabolic functions that occur in our bodies.[12,15]

Other sources that could hinder the utilization of EFAs are viruses, alcohol, insufficient zinc or insulin, excessive trans-fatty acid intake, and the aging process.

Uses:

Evening primrose oil has been shown to be useful in the following gynecological conditions:

- **Benign breast pain** (cyclic and non-cyclic mastalgia)[16]
- **Premenstrual Syndrome** (PMS)[17]

The most common use of EPO is in helping to control the symptoms of PMS. EPO has been shown to be effective in controlling abdominal and breast discomfort, irritability, depression and swollen joints. EPO has also been effective in the treatment of benign breast pain.[18,19] This is attributed to inhibition of prolactin due to a deficiency in prostaglandin E-1. In one study, EPO did not show any benefit against menopausal hot flushes,[20] but there are many anecdotal stories of its use for this purpose with some success.

Dosage:

For gynecological disorders, a dose of two to four grams daily in divided doses should be taken. This should continue for at least three to five menstrual cycles to see if it is effective. No adverse side effects have been seen with EPO. Since it is an oil, it would be advisable to take it with meals to help with its absorption.

REFERENCES: GYNECOLOGICAL DISORDERS

1.) Murray, Michael T
The Healing power of Herbs: The Enlightened Person's Guide to the Wonders of Medicinal Plants © 1992 pp 58-64

2.) Harada M, Suzuki M, Ozaki Y
Effect of Japanese Angelica root and peony root on uterine contraction in the rabbit in situ
J. Pharmacobiodyn 7 (5):304-11, 1984

3.) Tyler, Varro E
   Herbs of Choice: The Therapeutic Use of Phytomedicinals
   © 1994 pg. 136

4.) Lehmann-Willenbrock E, Riedel H.H.
   Zentralblatt fur Gynakologie
   110:611-618, 1988

5.) Bundesanzeiger (Cologne, Germany) January 5, 1989

6.) Duker EM, Kopanski L, Jarry H, Wuttke W
   Effects on extracts from Cimicifuga racemosa on gonadotropin release
   in menopausal women and ovariectomized rats
   Planta Med 1991 Oct; 57(5):420-424

7.) Weiss RF
   Herbal Medicine
   AbArcanum, Sweden 1988

8.) Amann W
   Removing an ostipation using Agnolyt
   Ther Gegenew 104 (9): 1263-1265 1965

9.) Reichert RD
   Phyto-estrogens
   Quart Rev Nat Med Spring 1994 pp 27-33

10.) Hobbs, Christopher
   Vitex
   In: Hoffmann, David, *The Herbalist* CD-ROM Version 2 © 1992
   Hopkins Technology, Hopkins, MN

11.) Mohr, H
   Clinical Investigations of means to increase lactation
   Dtsch Med Wschr 79 (41):1513-1516, 1954

12.) Leung, A
   Encyclopedia of Common Natural Ingredients, second edition
   New York, New York: John Wiley, 1996

13.) Brown, Donald J
   Herbal Prescriptions for Better Health
   © 1996 Prima Publishing, Rocklin, California 95677

14.) Harper, Harold A with Mayes, Peter
   "Metabolism of Lipids" in *Review of Physiological Chemistry*
   © 1971 Lange Medical Publications

15.) Oil of Evening Primrose (OEP) EPO
Review of Natural Products
© 1997 Monograph Date 8/97

16.) Belieu, RM
Mastodynia
Obstet Gynecol Clin North AM 1994 Sep; 21 (3): 461-477

17.) Campbell EM, Peterkin D, O'Grady K, Sanson-Fisher R
Premenstrual Symptoms in general practice patients
Prevalence and treatment
J Reprod Med 1997 Oct; 42 (10): 637-646

18.) Pye JK, Mansel RE, Hughes LE
Clinical experience of drug treatment for mastalgia
Lancet ii: 373-377, 1985

19.) Horrobin DF, Manku MS, et al
Abnormalities in plasma essential fatty acid levels in women with
premenstrual syndrome and with non-malignant breast disease
J Nutr Med 2: 259-264, 1991

20.) Chenoy R, Hussain S, Tayob Y, O'Brien PM, Moss MY, Morse PF
Effect of oral gamolenic acid from evening primrose oil on meno
pausal flushing
BMJ 1994 Feb 19; 308 (6927): 501-503

Hemorrhoids (external)

Hemorrhoids, or piles, are swollen veins around the anus that extend outward through the rectum. They can be caused by straining on defecation, especially if caused by constipation or poor diet. Pregnancy, standing or sitting for prolonged lengths of time, and lack of or too much exercise may also cause hemorrhoids. They may itch and cause a heavy feeling of discomfort in the rectum. Sometimes they bleed. If bleeding persists, medical help should be obtained.

Use:

- **Calendula**—Apply externally 4 times a day
- **Witch Hazel**—Apply externally 4 times a day

High-Blood Pressure

Hypertension, also known as high-blood pressure, is abnormally high pressure exerted on the walls of the arteries and veins that causes a constriction in the flow of blood. This can be caused by arteriosclerosis or atherosclerosis, which collectively form the basis of coronary-artery disease (CAD).

Blood pressure is usually read using an instrument called a sphygmomanometer. The reading consists of two numbers: the systolic pressure (the top number) refers to the pressure exerted when the heart pumps the blood out. The diastolic pressure (bottom number) refers to the pressure that is exerted to get the blood back to the heart. Because hypertension may have no signs or symptoms, a blood-pressure check should be performed every six months.

Use:

- **Dandelion**—500mg to 1000mg 3 times a day
- **Garlic**—3000mcg to 5000mcg (micrograms of allicin content) daily
- **Gugulipid**—25mg 3 times a day
- **Hawthorn**—80mg to 160mg 3 times a day

Hyperlipidemia (high cholesterol)

Hyperlipidemia, also known as high cholesterol, is usually caused by excessive consumption of fats in the diet. This can lead to atherosclerosis and coronary-artery disease (CAD).

Some cholesterol is necessary for normal body function. It is produced by the liver. Two types of cholesterol have significant importance. They are the high-density lipoproteins (HDL) which is the "good" cholesterol, and the low-density lipoproteins (LDL), the "bad" cholesterol. A total cholesterol reading is usually the addition of the HDL and LDL. A level of below 200 mg/dl is considered safe.

Use:

- **Garlic**—5000mcg (micrograms of allicin content) daily
- **Ginseng**—100mg to 500mg 3 times a day
- **Gugulipid**—25mg 3 times a day
- **Milk Thistle**—200mg 3 times a day

Immune System

We come in contact with infections every day of our lives. If our immune system is functioning properly, then we have no problem in combatting them even before we see any symptoms.

Many of the micro-organisms that exist on our planet are usually quite harmless. For example, as long as *E.coli* stays in the rectum it usually poses no problem. But if it enters by the mouth, then serious, if not sometimes fatal, results can occur.[1] Micro-organisms, whether bacteria or viruses, can enter the body in many ways—through the air, food, and skin[2] (Mom was right—wash those hands!). How our bodies deal with them is the function of our immune system.

Even though the immune system is a complex system of different mechanisms all working together to achieve one goal, it can be broken down into two categories: the cellular system and the humoral system.[2]

Cellular Immunity

Cellular immunity is composed of the macrophages and T-lymphocytes ("T" meaning that they are derived from the thymus gland).[3] These white blood cells are further broken down into T-cells and B-cells. T-cells include the T-helper cells and T-killer cells which produce tumor necrosis factor (TNF).

Humoral Immunity

Humoral immunity is derived from plasma cell production of antibodies (immunoglobulins). Plasma cells are derived from mature B-cells. There are five major immunoglobulins—IgG, IgM, IgA, IgD and IgE. (See figure 1.)

(Figure 1)

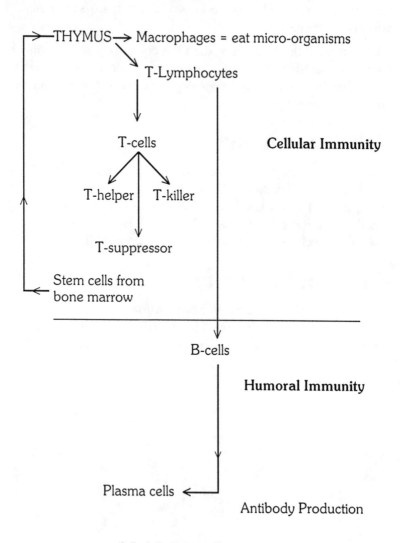

THYMUS → Macrophages = eat micro-organisms

T-Lymphocytes

T-cells   **Cellular Immunity**

T-helper | T-killer

T-suppressor

Stem cells from
bone marrow

B-cells

Humoral Immunity

Plasma cells ←

Antibody Production

(IgD, IgE, IgG, IgM, IgA)

Immune System Development

So what does all this mean?

It means that if there is a breakdown in one or more of these components, you are likely to come down with every cold or flu that you come in contact with. This could even include exposure to HIV.

Currently studies are being conducted on various plant derivatives for HIV treatment. The work is still in its early stages and therefore I cannot recommend any of them now. Let's hope that these plants may hold some answers to this disease.

Two herbs, echinacea and astragalus (*Astragalus membranaceus*) have been studied extensively. Both work to boost the immune system—but each in a slightly different manner. (Read more about these two herbs in Part Two.)

Use:

• **Astragalus**—500mg to 1000mg 3 times a day

• **Echinacea**—300mg 3 times a day

• **Garlic**—3000mcg (micrograms of allicin content) daily

• **Ginseng**—100mg to 500mg 3 times a day

REFERENCES: IMMUNE SYSTEM

1.) Lockie, Andrew
   The Family Guide to Homeopathy
   © 1993 Fireside Publishing, New York, New York 10020

2.) DiPiro JT, Talbert RL, Hayes PE, Yee GC, Possey LM
   Pharmacotherapy: A Pathophysiologic Approach Ch 57 pp. 845-855
   © 1989 Elsevier Science Publishing Co, New York, New York 10017

3.) Mills, Simon Y
   Out of the Earth: The Essential Book of Herbal Medicine pg. 68
   © 1991 Penguin Books, Viking Arkana, London

Insect Bites

Most insect bites are relatively harmless unless you are extremely sensitive to their venom. If this is the case, then it is advisable to carry an anaphylactic kit with you especially when insects are prevalent. The kit contains adrenaline, which can be injected to stop the progression of the reaction. A doctor's prescription is needed to obtain this product.

Use:
- **Aloe Vera**—Apply externally to affected area 3 to 4 times a day
- **Calendula**—Apply externally to affected area 3 to 4 times a day
- **Witch Hazel**—Apply externally to affected area 3 to 4 times a day

Insomnia

The body can go longer without food than it can without sleep. Insomnia is a pattern of sleeplessness. It does not include an occasional sleepless night or even a few nights in a row. It is persistent night after night.

Most people who suffer from insomnia do get some sleep but it just is not enough. They feel fatigued all the time. Insomnia can be caused by both mental and physical disorders. Pain, digestive disorders, caused by eating the wrong types of foods, and even drugs are just some of the physical problems that can cause sleeplessness. Anxiety and depression can also cause sleeplessness and fatigue. There are many physicians who specialize in sleep disturbances. Consult a doctor if insomnia persists more than a few weeks.

Use:

- **Chamomile**—500mg to 1000mg 1 hour before bedtime

- **Kava**—100mg to 200mg 1 hour before bedtime

- **Valerian**—300mg 1 hour before bedtime

Irritable Bowel Syndrome

Irritable bowel syndrome (IBS) can be a very distressing problem since modern medicine cannot find any anatomical reason for its existence. IBS presents itself with symptoms of stomachache, constipation, diarrhea, gas or bloating. It affects three times as many women as men.

Controlling the diet (especially if there is evidence of a food allergy), and stress management, seem to be the two best ways to treat this disorder. Fennel and enteric-coated peppermint oil tablets have been used in Europe with some success.

Use:

- **Chamomile**—500mg to 1000mg 3 to 4 times a day

- **Licorice** (DGL) —250mg to 500mg 3 times a day

- **Psyllium**—Use 1 tablespoonful of powder mixed with a full glass of water or juice daily

- **St. John's Wort**—300mg 3 times a day

- **Valerian**—100mg 3 times a day

Liver Disorders

The liver is the largest internal organ of the human body. It also can be considered as the great filter of the body. It is the only organ which can regenerate itself after injury or disease—provided that it has not gone too far.

The liver is a multifunctional organ, which metabolizes glucose and stores it as glycogen, stores all the fat-soluble vitamins (A, D, E and K), metabolizes fats and cholesterol, produces bile, filters toxins from foods, chemicals and drugs, and recycles old hemoglobin which carry red-blood cells (RBCs) just to name a few. A malfunction of any of its duties can cause many symptoms and illnesses that can range from mild to life-threatening.

Use:
• **Dandelion**—500mg to 1000mg 3 to 4 times a day
• **Milk Thistle**—200mg 3 times a day

Menopause

(Also see section under Gynecological Disorders.)

Let's start with diet. Soy, which most people in the United States do not understand or like, is loaded with the natural phytoestrogens of coumestrol, isoflavones, lignans and beta-sitosterol.[1,2] Phytoestrogens are derived from food or plants and bind to estrogen receptors in the body. They are *not* human or animal estrogens. Some produce estrogen-like functions while others may antagonize them. You might consider them as yin and yang. They try to balance and keep the body in a natural, steady state.

Some foods that you may want to include in your diet are tofu (in any way, shape or form), grains (especially oats, wheat, brown rice, corn), nuts (almonds and cashews), fruits and vegetables.[3,4] Some foods should be avoided as they may increase the many problems of menopause. Foods high in caffeine should be eliminated or drastically reduced. Carbonated beverages should also be avoided. Many soft drinks contain phosphorous, which causes the body to lose calcium.[3]

Excessive sugar intake should also be reduced. Sugar impairs the immune function and impedes the liver's ability to metabolize estrogen.[4] Excessive consumption of commercially raised meats, whether beef, chicken or pork, should also be reduced. This produces a higher saturated fat intake and decreased metabolism of estrogen.[5]

Women should also be taking some form of pro-biotic formula, which contains the "good" bacteria that inhabits our intestines. This will help with the metabolism and better utilization of estrogen. It should contain the strains of *Lactobacillus acidophilus* and *Bifidus* cultures.

• Exercise

As we age, both male and female lose bone density. We see less instances of osteoporosis in men than in women because males start out with a higher percentage of bone density. Moderate levels of weight-training exercises three to four times a week should be a part of every woman's therapy. It not only helps to improve bone mass, but also builds confidence and self-esteem.[6] There are also prescription medications available (e.g., Fosamax®) which can be used to help prevent bone-density loss, but they have their own side effects.

• Vitamins and Minerals

The next defensive position should be the use of vitamins and minerals. A good formula to use, includes:

• **Vitamin E**—400 to 800 IU (international units) daily—helps reduce hot flashes

• **Calcium**—1500mg daily helps maintain calcium balance. Calcium can only be absorbed if the stomach has an acid pH. High amounts of calcium carbonate raise the pH of the stomach and therefore less calcium is absorbed. This can be improved by taking it with meals or by drinking a small amount (1/4 teaspoonful) of pure apple cider vinegar in an ounce of warm water. A better source of calcium is microcrystalline calcium hydroxyapatite calcium (MCHC) or calcium citrate.[7]

• **Vitamin D**—400 to 800 units daily helps with absorption of calcium

• **Magnesium**—500mg to 750mg daily

• **Vitamin C**—1,000 to 2,000mg daily. Use with caution if you're susceptible to kidney stones. Vitamin C improves vitamin E absorption and decreases capillary fragility.

• Herbs that Help

• **Black Cohosh**—20mg to 60mg 3 times a day

• **Dong Quai**—500mg to 1000mg 2 to 3 times a day

• **Evening Primrose Oil**—500mg 3 to 4 times a day

• **Ginseng**—100mg to 500mg 3 times a day

• **Vitex Agnus Castus**—175mg daily

Menopause: If All Else Fails...

OK, you've gone the natural route but it seems that you still need some outside estrogen replacement. Granted, estrogen-replacement therapy does have some benefits—such as possibly decreasing the incidence of coronary-artery disease (CAD) by lowering cholesterol levels and helping to prevent the progression of osteoporosis, but which type of estrogen should a woman take?

There are also some risks involved, mainly the possible development of breast or uterine cancer. Many people mistakenly think estrogen is just, well, estrogen. Actually it is made up of three different types of estrogen called Estrone (E_1), Estradiol (E_2) and Estriol (E_3). Conjugated estrogens, such as Premarin, are not very well absorbed when taken orally. The liver destroys most of the forms of estrogen (E_1 and E_3) but leaves some of the Estradiol (E_2) in the form of 17 B-estradiol to be absorbed by the blood stream. Therefore higher doses of oral estrogen must be given to compensate for this effect.[8] Transdermal patches and creams eliminate some of this problem. The skin absorbs the medication directly into the blood stream and therefore can be given in lower dosages.

Unfortunately, E_1 and E_2 are the most potent forms of estrogen and the ones that may cause the risk factors to develop. There are many compounding pharmacies that can make any concentration of the E_1, E_2 and E_3 but the usual dose is 10 percent Estrone (E_1), 10 percent Estradiol (E2) and 80 percent Estriol (E_3).[9] In this manner, lesser amounts of E_1 and E_2 can be given while the amount of E_3 can be increased. E_3 can give the benefits of the estrogen but with less danger of developing breast or uterine cancer.[10] Recent investigation has also shown that estrogen may also work better when combined with progesterone to help balance the natural progesterone production. Natural progesterone also comes in a cream or transdermal patch or capsules. As you can see, there are many "natural" ways to enter into this cycle of life. It need not be entered with fear, but with the dignity and grace that mature womanhood brings.

REFERENCES: MENOPAUSE

1.) Burch, Beth
   Phytoestrogens and Menopause
   Eclectic Institute Inc. Sandy, Oregon 97055 1996

2.) Setchell KDR et al
   Nonsteroidal estrogens of dietary origin: possible roles in hormone
   dependent disease
   Am J Clin Nutr 1984 40:569-578

3.) Soffa M Ed, Virginia M
   Alternatives to Hormone Replacement for Menopause
   Alternative Therapies 1996 March Vol 2 No 2 pp 34-39

4.) Murray, Michael T
   Natural Alternatives to Over-the-counter and Prescription Drugs
   William Morrow: 1994 NY, NY

5.) Lark, Susan M
   *Dr. Susan Lark's Estrogen Decision Self Help Book: A Complete
   Guide for Relief of Menopausal Symptoms Through Hormone
   Replacement and Alternative Therapies*
   © 1996 Westchester Publishing Los Altos, California

6.) Shangold M
   Exercise in the menopausal woman
   Obstet Gynecol 1990:75 Suppl to No 40:538-578

7.) LaValle, James B
   Taking a natural approach to osteoporosis prevention
   Drug Store News Chain Pharmacy Sept 22, 1997 vol 7, No 10

8.) Davis KC, Goode J-V Robertson, Small RE
   Estrogen Replacement Therapy-Oral vs Transdermal
   US Pharmacist Sept 1997 Vol 22, No 9

9.) Petrin, Ron, personal communication

10.) Follingstad, A.H.
   Estriol, the forgotten estrogen?
   JAMA 239: 29-30 1978

Migraine Headaches

When a migraine develops, it can incapacitate its sufferer for four hours or up to four days. It usually develops either over or in back of the eye, or on the side of the head. Migraines can be either left or right sided or sometimes feel as if a tight band were being stretched around the head. Some migraines are accompanied by nausea and vomiting.

Migraines usually subside with rest and relaxation. They are more common in females than in males. Some migraine sufferers display auras before the full attack. These auras can be visual abnormalities (halos around lights, or bright colors, or spots dancing before the eyes), or physical disturbances in speech and sensation. The exact cause of migraine headaches is unknown but can be affected by diet, allergies, hormones, drugs, heredity and the environment.

Use:

- **Feverfew**—400mcg of standardized extract daily for prophylactic use
- **Ginkgo Biloba**—40mg 3 times a day
- **Ginger**—500mg to 1000mg 3 times a day
- **Valerian**—100mg 3 times a day

Nausea and Vomiting

One of the worst feelings that anyone can suffer through is that of nausea and vomiting. Though usually limiting, they could be symptoms of a larger disorder such as malnutrition, migraines, food poisoning or intestinal disorders. Nausea can be a symptom by itself or it can be accompanied with vomiting. If vomiting is also present and not controlled within 24 to 48 hours, seek professional help. Treatment is usually aimed at correcting the underlying disorder, but as long as there are no underlying disorders or any that are developing (e.g., dehydration), then letting it "run its course" is usually best.

Use:

- **Ginger**—500mg to 1000mg 4 times a day

Ophthalmic Disorders

It is said that "the eyes are the windows to the soul." But just as our souls sometimes become troubled, so can our eyes. Disturbances in these most precious organs can signal problems in other parts of the body. For example, watery, itchy eyes can signal an allergic reaction. Yellow eyes can signify liver or gall bladder problems.

By looking at the minute blood vessels and capillaries that surround the eye, a clinician can tell if a person is having problems with his or her blood pressure.

Following are a number of common eye problems and some natural products that can provide solutions to possible relief.

Cataracts

In one study, 50 patients were given an extract of bilberry and vitamin E. It stopped the progression of senile cortical cataracts in 97 percent of the patients (reference 7 under bilberry in Part Two, The Healing Herbs).

Glaucoma

Bilberry has also shown promise in the treatment and prevention of glaucoma because of its effects on the collagen structure of the eye. Collagen provides tensile strength and integrity to the tissues of the eye, which may result in decreased intraocular pressure (IOP) (reference 8 under bilberry in Part Two.)

Night Vision

Bilberry's ophthalmic applications extend to improvement of people who have difficulty with night vision (read the RAF story under bilberry, Part Two). It appears that the anthocyanosides speed up the regeneration of the rods in the retina of the eye. The rods are the part of the eye that helps us to see at night and help the eye adapt to varying intensities of light. In one study, patients were given a combination of bilberry (400mg a day) and beta-carotene (20mg a day) and showed an improvement in their night vision and light adaptation. (Reference 11 under bilberry in Part Two).

Dosage:

A standardized extract of the anthocyanoside content between 15 percent to 25 percent should be given. This equates to 80 to 160mg 3 times a day. No adverse side effects have been shown.

Caution:

Bilberry may affect clotting times due to its decrease in platelet aggregation (reference 12 under bilberry, Part Two).

Macular Degeneration

Diabetics, especially elderly diabetics, whether on insulin or not, are much more susceptible to the degeneration of the arteries and veins that carry blood to the eyes. When these tiny capillaries become blocked, senile macular degeneration or retinal insufficiency can develop. At the end of one study (reference 17 under gingko biloba in Part Two), visual acuity (how clearly we see) and visual field (how much we see), as measured by funduscopic examination had improved by almost four times (2.3 diopters) over the placebo group (0.6 diopters).

Dosage:

Extract of gingko biloba's (EGb) beneficial effects can usually be seen if it is taken consistently for at least four to six months. The recommended dosage of the standardized 24 percent extract is a daily dose of 120mg to 240mg in divided doses of either two to three times daily (40mg to 80mg) with meals. The 240mg is usually reserved for cerebral insufficiencies. Because so much of the plant is used to achieve a 24 percent extract, the beneficial effects of ginkgo cannot be achieved by drinking a tea (reference 18 under gingko biloba section in Part Two).

Gingko Biloba Cautions and Side Effects

Due to its PAF (platelet-activating factor) effects, EGb should be used with caution in patients receiving anti-coagulant therapy. This would include both warfarin compounds and aspirin. Some people have also experienced mild gastrointestinal problems (reference 19 under gingko biloba in Part Two).

Peptic Ulcer and Reflex Disorders

Peptic ulcer disease, also known as PUD, is a generic term that is used to describe all types of ulcers (duodenal and gastric) that occur in the upper gastro-intestinal tract. In most cases, the body's natural defense mechanism of secreting mucous in the GI tract to protect itself against the hydrochloric acid that is secreted and needed for proper digestion of food does not function properly. Many factors contribute to ulcer formation including age (usually over 40 years of age), genetics (family history), overuse of aspirin and other non-steroidal, anti-inflammatory agents such as ibuprofen and naproxen, steroids and smoking.

There is also evidence that some ulcers may be associated with a bacterium known as *Helicobacter pylori*. A short treatment of antibiotics has been successful in some patients in eliminating this bacteria. Gastroesophageal reflux disorder (GERD) can also pose problems for many people. Although not considered specifically as an ulcer, GERD occurs when the contents of the stomach reflex upwards into the esophagus. Most people will complain of heartburn especially while lying down.

In some cases, GERD has been shown to cause asthma attacks when the acid contents of the stomach makes its way up the esophagus to the oral cavity, then travels back down the throat and irritates the bronchial tract.

Use:

- **Chamomile**—500mg to 1000mg 3 times a day
- **Deglycyrrhizinated Licorice** (DGL) —250mg to 500mg 4 times a day
- **Slippery Elm**—300mg to 500mg 3 times a day
- **Valerian** (for stress management) —100mg 3 times a day

Peripheral Vascular Disorders

Intermittent claudication, which can best be described as cramping and pain in the lower legs (especially the calf) when walking, is due primarily to poor peripheral circulation in the veins.

EGb (extract gingko biloba) has been shown to be effective in this disorder (reference 15 under gingko biloba in Part Two). It has also been shown to be effective in other circulatory disorders such as Raynaud's disease (cold hands and feet). (See reference 16 under gingko biloba in Part Two).

Premenstrual Syndrome

(See also Gynecological Disorders)

Premenstrual syndrome (PMS) describes an array of problems both physical and psychological, which affects women about one to two weeks before menses and usually disappears one or two days after menstruation begins.

Dysmenorrhea (painful menstruation) usually replaces PMS after menses begins. Most women go through minor changes, but usually these symptoms are not debilitating. Some of these symptoms may include nausea, depression, anxiety, water retention, cramps, skin eruptions and breast tenderness.

Use:

- **Dong Quai**—500mg to 1000mg 2 to 3 times a day
- **Evening Primrose Oil** (EPO) —500mg to 1000mg 3 times a day
- **Ginseng**—100mg to 500mg 3 times a day
- **Valerian**—100mg 3 times a day

Raynaud's Disease

If you describe the symptoms of Raynaud's disease to anyone living in cold climates, you may be surprised to find out that everyone will admit to having it. Hopefully this is not the case since advanced Raynaud's includes the formation of external ulcers of the fingers and toes caused by poor circulation.

Mild cases of Raynaud's can best be described as hypersensitivity of the extremities to cold due to poor circulation and lack of oxygen. This can be caused by improper diet, lack of exercise, excessive smoking and even some prescription drugs known as beta-blockers which are uses to treat high-blood pressure.

Use:

- **Capsaicin**—Apply externally up to 5 times a day. Avoid facial and eye contact.
- **Garlic**—3000mcg to 5000mcg (micrograms of allicin content) daily

- **Gingko biloba**—40mg to 80mg 3 times a day
- **Ginger**—500mg to 1000mg 4 times a day

Respiratory Tract Disorders

(Also see the section on Asthma)

A discussion about medicinal herbal therapy would not be complete without references to the management of the mucous membranes that make up the respiratory system. Herbal materia medica, from any system that uses plants exclusively for their treatment regimen—Aruveydic, Western herbalism or TCM (Traditional Chinese Medicine)—abound with singular and combination products to treat problems that are associated with the respiratory tract, no matter if they are caused by allergies or infections. Although you may find the following herbs used in combination with each other, I have chosen to list them separately so that you may understand their usage more clearly. My best advice would be to purchase these herbs in a liquid form (if available) so that a tea can be prepared. Not only is there the benefit of a more rapid absorption into the body, but also the warmth of the liquid itself will have a soothing and relaxing effect on the respiratory tract. Since tinctures come in varying strengths and potencies, follow the recommended dosage schedule of whichever product you purchase.

Helpful Herbs:

- **Slippery Elm** *(Ulmus rubra and U. fulva)*

The inner bark of the tree is used medicinally. The tree is found in the central and northern USA. It is a soothing demulcent (a demulcent is a substance that can soothe and protect irritated mucous membranes of the respiratory tract), especially for the throat. Slippery elm is rich in polysaccharide (sugar) molecules which expand when they come in contact with moisture. Slippery elm is sometimes an effective antitussive.[1,2] You can find it as a tea or commercially prepared lozenges. Both forms can be used at the same time. Each has a different advantage. Slippery elm tea not only soothes the respiratory tract, but the warmth of the liquid also helps relax the throat and bronchial tree. The lozenges offer the convenience of portability.

Use: Helps soothe any irritation of the throat or larynx.

• **Marshmallow Root** (*Althea officinalis*)

Another excellent demulcent is marshmallow root. This is a good example of how different parts of the same plant are used for different systems. The leaves are used more for the mucous membranes of the upper respiratory tract while the roots are used more specifically for the digestive system. Marshmallow root has excellent properties as a soothing throat herb and as an expectorant.[3]

Use: Helps soothe any irritation of the throat and larynx.

• **Eyebright** (*Euphrasia officinalis*)

Eyebright, as its name implies, can be used for any problems associated with watery and irritated eyes. It has been helpful in the treatment of allergies and conjunctivitis.[3] It can also be used externally as a cold compress on the eyes. The herb is meant to be taken internally or used externally as a compress. It is *never to be used as an eye drop.*

Use: Decreases the hyperactivity of the mucous membranes of the eyes, nose, throat and ears. Excellent to use for watery and itchy eyes, conjunctivitis, sinusitis and rhinitis, especially when caused by allergies.

• **Mullein** (*Verbascum thapus*)

Mullein is another wonderful herb that is especially useful for the upper portion of the respiratory tract (larynx and trachea). It is an ideal remedy for inflammation of the throat, especially when someone has a dry, nonproductive cough. It has also been shown to stimulate fluid production and thus facilitate expectoration.[3] Mullein will work best to soothe a throat that has been irritated by excessive coughing if the fluid extract is made into a tea and mixed with a teaspoonful of pure honey or pure maple syrup. The warmth of the liquid will not only help soothe and relax the mucous membranes, but also help the body absorb the herbs into the system. The flowers and leaves hold the medicinal properties of the plant.

Uses: Irritated throat caused by or with a nonproductive hacking cough. May also be useful as an expectorant.

• **Nettles** (*Urtica dioica*)

Nettles, also known as stinging nettles, are known to many a gardener as a common weed. I do not advise that you go out into the back yard and start picking the leaves off this plant. The leaves are prickly and can cause a rash if not handled properly. (The medical term *urticaria* is directly translated from "Urtica" or nettle rash.)[6] I will limit the use of nettles to the treatment of allergic rhinitis, although nettles has been used to treat arthritis and gout by removing uric acid and probably removing other acid metabolites from the body via its mild diuretic properties.[4]

Stinging nettles rot has also shown some promise in the treatment of Benign Prostatic Hyperplasia (BPH),[5-7] but mainly we'll discuss the value of this herb's treatment of allergic rhinitis (runny nose caused by allergies). Nettles stabilize the mast cell and thus prevent the cell wall from breaking and releasing the substances that cause the reaction.[8] Mast cells are curious structures that are scattered throughout connective tissue. They contain large amounts of histamine and other inflammatory compounds (i.e., leucotrienes). When the cell wall breaks, these compounds are released into the blood stream and cause all sorts of problems.

The drug cromolyn works on this same principle.[9-10] Studies have shown that 300mg in capsule form given twice daily for seven days will usually identify the population that will derive the most benefit.[11]

Uses: Allergic rhinitis and adjuvant treatment of BPH. (Adjuvant is any type of therapy—medicinal, physical or psychological—that works with other therapies to hasten the healing process.)

• Quercetin

Quercetin is best described as a flavonoid. Flavonoids, sometimes known as bioflavonoids, are naturally occurring antioxidants that are contained in many fruits, plants and vegetables. The bioflavonoids act synergistically with Vitamin C. Quercetin, which can be found in most plants especially in citrus fruits (concentrated mostly in the white pulp under the skin—the stuff nobody eats!), has been found to be useful in the treatment and prevention of allergic reactions by stabilizing the mast cell wall, thereby preventing the release of histamine and other inflammatory compounds that are contained within the cell.[9-10]

Quercetin can be found singularly or in combination with bromelain, an enzyme obtained from the pineapple which also aids in the reduction of the inflammatory process.[12-14] If you purchase a product that contains both quercetin and bromelain, make sure that you take it between meals. Bromelain is an enzyme, which, if taken with food, will help more with digestion than with inflammation. In one study,[15] 500mg of bromelain three times a day between meals was used to relieve musculoskeletal injuries (pulled and strained muscles and ligaments) with great success.

A daily dose of 500mg of quercetin in capsule form, three to four times a day is usually sufficient to produce a satisfactory response. I have also used this dose to alleviate arthritic, sports and muscle pain with great success.

Uses: Good for allergic reactions and as an anti-inflammatory

USE WITH CAUTION

Due to their many contra-indications and side effects, the following herbs should only be used under the supervision of a trained clinician:

• Ephedra *(Ephedra sinica)*

Ephedra, also known by its Chinese name ma huang, has been used for centuries in the treatment of asthma. Ephedra is the plant and ephedrine is one of the alkaloids that is derived from the plant. In addition to ephedrine, several other alkaloids, including pseudoephedrine, norephedrine, norpseudoephedrine, etc. are contained in various species of ephedra.[17] Because of its actions on both the alpha and beta-adrenergic cells, ephedra can cause nervousness, irritability, increased heart rate, dilated pupils, nausea and vomiting. Therefore people with heart conditions, hypertension, thyroid problems, diabetes, glaucoma or prostate problems should not use it since exacerbation of symptoms could occur.

• Lobelia

Lobelia inflata, also known as Indian tobacco and pukeweed, is another herb that needs to be approached with caution. Although it has been used to treat bronchial conditions, it works as an expectorant (hence the name pukeweed). Lobeline, the active ingredient, has similar properties of nicotine but is less potent.[19] Lobeline has been used as a smoking deterrent in place of the nicotine patches and gum. Although toxic reactions for an overdose of lobelia are rare, it can cause the same reactions as nicotine poisoning (nausea, vomiting, blurred vision and confusion) if taken in high doses. If lobelia is used in a combination product with other herbs that affect the respiratory system, it should pose no problem.

REFERENCES: RESPIRATORY DISORDERS

1.) Tyler, Varro E
      Herbs of Choice: The Therapeutic Use of
      Phytomedicinals
      © 1994 Hawthorn Press Inc, Binghamton, New York 13904

2.) Lawrence Review of Natural Products
March 1991

3.) Hoffmann, David
The Herbalist
CD-ROM Version 2 © 1992 Hopkins Technology, Hopkins, MN

4.) Mills, Simon Y.
Out of the Earth: The Essential Book of Herbal Medicine
© 1991 Penguin Books, Viking Arkana, London

5.) Bundesanzeiger (Cologne, Germany)
January 5, 1989; March 6, 1990

6.) Lichius JJ, Muth C
The inhibiting effects of Urtica diorica root extracts on experimentally
induced prostatic hyperplasia in the mouse
Planta Med 1997 Aug; 63(4): 307-310

7.) Vahlensieck W Jr, Fabricius PG, Hell W
Drug therapy of benign prostatic hyperplasia
Fortschr Med 1996 Nov 10; 114(31):407-411

8.) Morningstar, Amanda and Gagnon, Daniel O
Breathe Free: Nutritional and Herbal Care for Your Respiratory System
Lotus Press, Wilmot, WI 53192 © 1991

9.) Ogasawara H, Middelton E Jr
Effect of selected flavonoids on histamine release (HR) and hydrogen
peroxide (H2O2) generation by human leucocytes
J Allergy Clinical Immunol 75:184, 1985

10.) Beck WS
Human Design
Harcourt Brace Jovanovich Inc, NY © 1971

11.) Mittman P
Randomized, double blind study of freeze-dried Urtica
dioica in the management of allergic rhinitis
Planta Med 56:44-47 1990

12.) Welton AF, Tobias LD, Fiedler-Nagy C, et al
Effects of flavonoids on arachidonic acid metabolism
Prog Clin Biol Res 213: 231-242; 1986

13.) Ryan RE
A double-blind clinical evaluation of bromelains in the treatment of
acute sinusitis
Headache 7 (1): 13-17, 1967

14.) Taub, SJ
The use of bromelains in sinusitis: A double-blind clinical evaluation
Eye Ear Nose Throat Mon 46 (3): 361-362 passim 1967

15.) Masson, M
Bromelain in the treatment of blunt injuries to the musculoskeletal system
Fortschr Med 1995; 113 (19): 303-306

16.) Tyler, Varro E
Herbs of Choice: The Therapeutic Use of Phytomedicinals, pp. 88-89
© 1994 Hawthorn Press Inc, Binghamton, New York 13904-1580

17.) Mansuri, S, Kelkar V, Jindal M
Some pharmacological characteristics of ganglionic activity of lobeline
Arzneim Forsch 23: 1271-1275, 1973

Tinnitus

As one person described it, tinnitis is "like hearing church bells in your head 24 hours a day." Persistent ringing in the ears or other noises can also be present. It may be caused by foreign objects in the ears, aging or medications, especially high doses of aspirin or other drugs called salicylates. Some cases are more pronounced during the winter months when the air is dry and cold.

Use:
• **Ginkgo Biloba**—40mg to 80mg 3 times a day

Travel Sickness

We once had a dog who hated riding in a car. The first day we brought her home, she was carsick. She apparently never forgot the feelings that accompany travel/motion sickness—and was reluctant to ever ride in the car again.

Whether you're on a plane or train or in a car or boat, any mild disturbance of the middle ear may result in a pale complexion, cold and clammy skin, nausea or vomiting. Reading while in motion or sharply turning the head can send conflicting messages from the eyes to the brain which can trigger the reactions producing those unpleasant symptoms.

Use:

• **Ginger**—500mg to 1000mg 4 times a day

Urinary Tract Infections

Although herbal remedies have been taken for the treatment of urinary tract disorders, phytotherapy should not be the only method of treatment. Problems affecting the urethra (urethritis), the bladder (cystitis), and the kidney (pyelonephritis) area are a much too serious set of disorders to rely solely on the use of plants. Plant therapy should and can be used as adjuvant (complementary) therapy in both the prophylaxis and treatments of any disorder involving the urinary tract.

Cystitis is an inflammation of the bladder caused by bacteria, usually *Escherichia coli*. If it is not treated *E.coli* can travel up the ureters and into the kidneys causing the more serious problems of pyelonephritis. The self-treatment of a bladder infection should not be taken lightly. As seen, it can progress to a more serious situation. Recurrence can be held to a minimum with herbal preventive measures.

Use:

• **Cranberry**—500mg to 1500mg of concentrate (capsules) 3 times a day with a full glass of water

• **Echinacea**—30 drops of a standardized tincture or 300mg 4 times a day

• **Goldenseal**—250mg to 500mg 4 times a day

- **Uva ursi**—500mg 4 times a day. Not to be used for more than 3 days. An elaboration of these herb treatments follows.

Helpful Herbs:

• Cranberry (*Vaccinium macrocarpon*)

One of the better known adjuvant therapies to help with urinary tract infections is the cranberry. The Pilgrims learned about the properties of this plant from the American Indians. The Penobscot Tribe of Maine used cranberries for the treatment of gravel and other kidney and bladder troubles (gravel in the urinary tract was the name given to what is now called kidney stones).[1]

Mechanism of Action:

Many people are aware of the benefits of drinking cranberry juice in order to acidify the urine and thus inhibit the growth of *E.coli*, which is the major cause of more complicated urinary tract infections (UTI). But the patient would have to drink a quart of juice at a time!

This would be a Herculean task for anyone and, therefore, the rate of success and compliance would be negative, not to mention the amount of sugar that is in the disguise of corn syrup that is used in the manufacturing process in order to make the cranberries more palatable. (Eating raw cranberries will give your mouth the same response as trying to eat a lemon!)

Although cranberries do acidify the urine, studies were done to show that this was not the only method of action.[2-5] It seems that cranberry juice inhibits the adhesion or sticking of *E.coli* to the mucous membrane of the urethra and bladder.[6] If treatment were combined with a sufficient amount of water intake (six eight-ounce glasses daily), then the *E.coli* would be flushed from the system and would not have enough time to infect the mucosa and cause problems.

Dosage:

As stated earlier, trying to drink 32 ounces of anything, let alone cranberry juice at one time, would be difficult for anyone. Luckily, cranberry concentrate capsules do exist and can be taken instead of drinking all that fluid. One to three capsules of cranberry-concentrate capsules (500 to 1500mg) should be taken three times daily with a sufficient fluid intake (which can include water and cranberry concentrate). Do not use the "cocktail" type drinks since they contain too much sugar.

Other Uses:

Since cranberry inhibits *E.coli's* ability to stick to the urinary mucosa, it may be beneficial in the treatment of other disorders involving the urinary tract system such as:

• Catheterized patients

• Nursing home residents, especially if they have an indwelling catheter

• Reduction and prevention in kidney stone formation due to the higher acidity of the urine

Miscellaneous Herbs for UTI

The following is a list of herbs that have been used in the treatment of UTIs:

• Berberis, echinacea, goldenseal, and Oregon grape

This variety of herbs can be used for their mild antimicrobial actions.

• Celery

Yes, good old-fashioned celery can be used as a diuretic. This can be obtained from either capsules or by making your own by using a juicer.

• Marshmallow root and mullein

These two herbs can help soothe the irritated mucous membranes of the urinary tract.

• Yarrow

Yarrow can be used effectively as a urinary antiseptic.

• Uva Ursi (*Arctostaphylos*)

Uva ursi, also known as bearberry, has been used as a urinary antiseptic. Its mechanism of action is in its arbutin content. Arbutin is hydrolized to hydroquinone.[7] But in order for it to work, the urine must be alkaline (pH above 8).[8] This would be impractical in most cases and would negate the effects of other herbs which rely on an acid medium.

• Goldenrod (*Solidago*)

Goldenrod has been used in Europe as a diuretic. Don't confuse the goldenrod with what some people also call ragweed (*Ambrosia*).

No complications or contraindications have been observed for either cranberry or the other herbs that are mentioned.

REFERENCES: URINARY TRACT DISORDERS

1.) Chief Needahbeh
"Medicine plants of our Maine Indians" as told to Lucinda Lombard, Circa 1934

2.) Bodel PT, Cotran R, Kass EH
Cranberry juice and antibacterial action of hippuric acid
J Lab Clin Med 54: 881-888 1959

3.) Moen DV
Observations on the effectiveness of cranberry juice in urinary tract infections
Wis Med J 61: 282-283 1962

4.) Papas PN, Brusch CA, Ceresia GC
Cranberry juice in the treatment of urinary tract infections
Southwest Med 47: 17-20 1966

5.) Walker EB, Barney DP, Mickelsen JN, Walton RJ, Michelsen RA Jr

Cranberry concentrate: UTI prophylaxsis
J Fam Pract 1997 Aug; 45(2): 167-168 (letter)

6.) Ofek I, Goldhar J, Sharon N
Anti-Escherichia coli adhesion activity of cranberry and blueberry juices
Adv Exp Med Biol 1996; 408: 179-183

7.) Mills, Simon Y
Out of the Earth: The Essential Book of Herbal Medicine, pg. 282
© 1991 Penguin Books, Viking Arkana, London

8.) Tyler, Varro E
Herbs of Choice: The Therapeutic Use of Phytomedicinals, pg. 79
© 1994 Hawthorn Press Inc., Binghamton, New York 13904-1580

Vertigo

Vertigo is usually caused by a disturbance in equilibrium. Sometimes it is known as "dizziness." Unlike travel or motion sickness, vertigo sufferers feel that the room is tilted or spinning. They may be standing upright, but to them things seem to be at a 45-degree angle. This can produce problems even in the simple task of just standing upright.

Use:

• **Ginger**—500mg to 1000mg every 4 hours

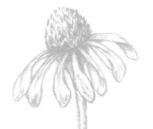

PART TWO

THE
HEALING
HERBS

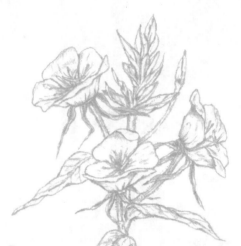

*Better to use medicines at the outset
than at the last moment.*

~Publius Syrus 42 BC.

Astragalus

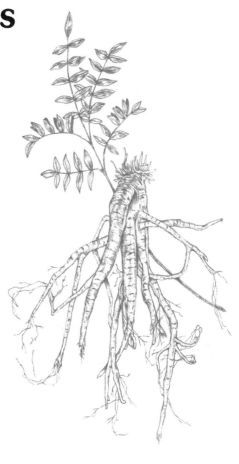

Astragalus (*Astraga-lus membranaceus*), also known as *huang qi* in Chinese, is an herb, which is more common to Traditional Chinese Medicine (TCM) than to Western herbalism. It was, and still is, used as a tonic mixed with other herbs for general health.

Astragalus is a member of the "pea" family (Legumiosae) or "vetch," hence it is also known as milk vetch. Do not confuse the *membranaceus* with other species of astragalus like the *trichopodus* or *gummifera*. The *membranaceus* is the one that is used medicinally. The *gummifera*, also known as tragacanth is used as a thickening agent in making candy, pharmaceuticals and cosmetics. The root contains its medicinal properties.

Mechanism of Action:

Like echinacea, astragalus is composed of large polysaccharide (sugar) molecules. One of them, called astragalan B, binds to the outer cell wall of bacteria and viruses, and therefore interferes with its metabolism. Astragalus has also been shown to stimulate T-cell functions and activity.[1] One study has also shown that astragalus increased natural killer cell activity (NK) in patients suffering from viral Coxsackie B myocarditis infection.[2]

Uses:

In Traditional Chinese Medicine, astragalus is used to strengthen the "Wei Qi," or immune system. Qi or chi (pronounced "chee") is loosely translated as "life force." Astragalus, like echinacea, can be used in most instances where the immune system needs some help. It can be used to treat and prevent colds or the flu. But one of its more promising attributes seems to be in its ability to help the immune system recover at a more rapid pace when subjected to chemotherapy or radiation therapy. In one case, 54 patients with small-cell lung cancer (SCLC) were treated with radiotherapy and chemotherapy, which consisted of the drugs vincristine, cyclophosphamide, methotrexate, and carmustine. By combining the different therapies (chemo, radiation, and herbal), some of the patients gained anywhere from three to 17 years in survival time.[3]

In another study, a high molecular weight polysaccaride fraction obtained from astragalus was combined with recombinant interleukin-2 (rIL-2). The results showed that the astragalus potentiated the rIL-2's ability to produce lymphokine-activated killer cells (LAK). It did this so well, that a 10-fold less dose of rIL-2 was needed. This in turn lead to fewer side effects (capillary leakage, gastrointestinal, visual disturbances, and fluid imbalances), not to mention cost.[4]

Dosage:

Take 500mg to 1000mg 3 to 4 times a day with food
Astragalus comes in both capsule and liquid form. Follow the directions on the bottle.

REFERENCES: ASTRAGALUS

1.) Chu D-T, et al
Immunotherapy with Chinese medicinal herbs. I. Immune restoration of local xenogenic graft-versus-host reaction in cancer patients by

fractioned Astragalus membranaceus in vitro
J Clin Lab Immunol 25: 119-123, 1988

2.) Yang YZ, et al
Effect of Astragalus membranaceus on natural killer cell activity and
induction with coxsakie B viral myocarditis
Chin Med J 103 (4): 304-307, 1990

3.) Cha RJ, Zeng DW, Chang QS
"Non-surgical treatment of small cell lung cancer with chemo-radio-
immunotherapy and traditional Chinese medicine"
Chung-Hua-Nei-Ko-Tsa-Chih (Chinese Journal of Internal Medicine)
7/94 33 (7): 462-466

4.) Wang Y, Qian X, Hadley HR, et al
Phytochemicals potentiate interleukin-2 generated lymphokine-activated
killer cell cytotoxicity against murine renal cell carcinoma
Mol Biother 4: pp. 143-146, 1992

Bilberry

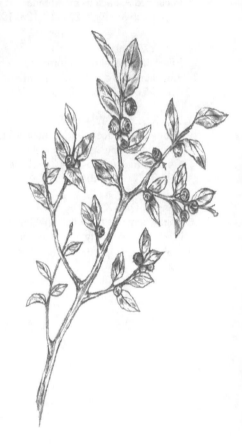

B ilberry (*Vaccinium myrtillus*) is also known as European blueberry. Although they are from the same family (Ericaceae), it should not be confused with *Vaccinium corymbosum*, the American blueberry.[1] The ripened berries and the leaves are used medicinally, but exert different effects. The leaves are used in the same manner as uva ursi (i.e., urinary tract infections).[2] We will focus on the medicinal use and properties of the fruit.

Mechanism of Action:

Bilberry contains potent bioflavonoids especially the anthocyanosides.[3,4] These bioflavonoids act as potent anti-oxidants and help to counteract the damaging effects of free radicals. (Free radicals are molecules, which have an uneven amount of electrons. They try to balance themselves by "stealing" electrons from stable molecules.)

Bilberry's anthocyanosides stabilize connective tissue by increasing the integrity of the collagen matrix, increasing the production of collagen and by preventing the destruction of collagen connective tissue around blood vessels. Collagen is a fibrous structural protein of the skin, tendons, ligaments, cartilage muscles and other connective tissues of the body. It is the most common protein of the body. It is also dispersed in the vitreous liquid of the eye to form a gel that helps maintain the proper stiffness and shape of the eye.

Uses:

Because of its potent antioxidant effect, bilberry has been used to treat everything from urinary tract infections to diarrhea, but it is in the treatment of ophthalmic and diabetic problems that it has met with the most success.

There is an anecdotal story of the Royal Air Force (RAF) pilots back in World War II, who noticed that their vision, especially night vision, improved after consuming bilberry jam before a bombing raid.[5,6] This warranted further investigation of how bilberry affected vision.

Ophthalmic Disorders

Cataracts

In one study, 50 patients were given an extract of bilberry and Vitamin E. It stopped the progression of senile cortical cataracts in 97 percent of the patients.[7]

Glaucoma

Bilberry has also shown promise in the treatment and prevention of glaucoma because of its effects on the collagen structure of the eye. Collagen provides tensile strength and integrity to the tissues of the eye, which may result in decreased intraocular pressure (IOP).[8]

Diabetes

Diabetics are more prone to develop cataracts due to the decrease in microcirculation in the capillaries. Diabetic cataracts develop from excessive absorption of sorbitol in the lens of the eye.[9]

In a study done on patients with different types of visual problems which include diabetic retinopathy, retinitis pigmentosa, macular degeneration and hemorrhagic retinopathy due to an-

ticoagulant therapy, all the patients had a reduction in hemor-
rhage and an improvement in circulation[10] while using bilberry.

Night Vision

Bilberry also improves the condition of those suffering from
difficulty with night vision (remember the RAF story). It appears that the anthocyanosides speed up the regeneration of
the rods in the retina of the eye. The rods are the part of the eye
that helps us see at night, and helps the eye adapt to varying
intensities of light. In one study, patients given a combination of
bilberry (400mg a day) and beta-carotene (20mg a day), showed
an improvement in their night vision and light adaptation.[11]

Dosage:

A standardized extract of the anthocyanoside content between
15 percent to 25 percent should be given. This equates to 80 to
160mg three times a day. No adverse side effects have been
shown. Take it with food.

Caution:

Bilberry may affect clotting times due to its decrease in platelet aggregation.[12]

REFERENCES: BILBERRY

1.) Tyler, Varro E
   Herbs of Choice: The Therapeutic Use of Phytomedicinals
   © 1994 Hawthorn Press Inc., Binghamton, New York 13904-1580

2.) Grieve, Mrs. M.
   A Modern Herbal
   New York, NY: Dover Publications, © 1971.

3.) Anderson O.M.
   Anthocyanins in fruits of Vaccinium uliginosum L. (bog whortleberry)
   J Food Sci 1987 52: 665-666, 680

4.) Baj A, Bombarelli E, et al
   Qualitative and quantitative evaluation of *Vaccinium myrtillus* anthocyanins by high-resolution gas chromatography and high performance
   liquid chromatography

J Chromatography 1983 279: 365-372

5.) Brown, Donald J
Herbal Prescriptions for Better Health
© 1996 Prima Publishing, Rocklin, California 95677

6.) Werbach, Melvin R
Nutritional Influences on Illness
© 1996 Second Edition, Third Line Press, Tarzana, California 91356

7.) Bravetti, G
Preventive medical treatment of senile cataract with Vitamin E and
anthocyanosides: clinical evaluation
Ann Ottalmol Clin Ocul 1989 115:109

8.) Murray, Michael
The Healing Power of Herbs
© 1992 Prima Publishing, Rocklin, California 95677

9.) Varma SD, Mizuno A, Kinoshita JH
Diabetic cataracts and flavonoids
Science 1977 195:87-89

10.)Scharrer A, Ober M
"Anthocyanosides in the treatment of retinopathies"
Klin Monastbl Augenheilkd 1981 178:386-389

11.)Fiorni G, Biancacci A, Graziano FM
Perimetric and adaptometric modifications of anthocyanosides and
beta-carotene
Ann Ottal Clin Ocul 1965 91:371-386

12.)Zaragoza F, Iglesias I, Benedi J
Comparison of thrombocyte anti-aggregant effects of anthocyanosides
with those of other agents
Arch Pharmacol 1985 11:183-188

Chamomile

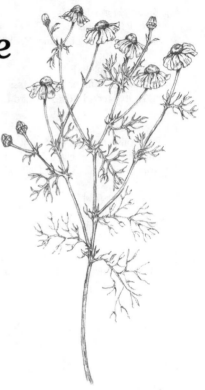

*M*atricaria recutita, also known as German chamomile, is a true herb in the sense that it has graced many a garden since the times of the Pharaohs of ancient Egypt.

The name is from a Greek derivation of which describes its aromatic fragrance—*Kamal* (on the ground) and *melon* (an apple).[1] There are many different forms and plant species of chamomile but only the German *(Matricaria)* and another called Roman chamomile (*Anthemus nobilis*), are the preferred species used medicinally, especially the German species which is seen mostly in the United States.[2,3] The flowers are used medicinally.

Mechanism of Action:

The active ingredients of chamomile are composed of the volatile oils alpha-bisabolol and bisabolol oxide, and the flavonoids apigenin, luteolin and quercetin. Apigenin has been shown to have anxiolytic (relaxing) activity without the sedative effects associated with the benzodiazepines (Valium®, Xanax® and Librium®)[4] while bisabolol affects the gastro-intestinal tract. When distilled, the oil has a deep blue color.[5,6] This is a good example of a plant with many constituents which all act together to achieve the intended response.

94

Uses:

Chamomile can be used in the following conditions:

- Anxiety
- Colic
- Flatulence
- Indigestion
- Insomnia
- Intestinal cramps
- Irritable bowel syndrome
- Irritated skin
- Stress
- Teething

Actually the list could continue. Chamomile was voted "Medicinal Plant of the Year" for 1987 in Germany.[7,8] But if it helps to narrow it down, just remember to use chamomile anywhere that you need to relax the nervous system, or for use as a carminative (substance that promotes the elimination of intestinal gas) to enhance the digestive system.

Chamomile can be used to relieve tension caused by stress and to help relieve digestive problems that may be caused by the stress (flatulence, intestinal cramps and indigestion). A cup of tea before bed will usually help relax the body before sleep. The tea may also be taken during the day, which will relieve stress and act as an anti-spasmodic in the digestive tract. A preparation of the tea may also be given to children who are teething and/or colic. By putting the child to bed with a bottle of chamomile tea (instead of milk or juice, which contain sugar), the baby will be able to sleep (not to mention the parents!).

A wet compress or ointment of chamomile can also be used for many skin irritations including eczema and other skin inflammations.[9] A few drops of the pure oil in baby's bath will also help diaper rash (the oil should be used **only externally**).[10] Chamomile comes in many forms including tea, capsules, tincture, elixir and even fresh or dried flowers. Use whichever is to your liking. If you purchase the capsules, you can always break them open and use them to prepare a tea. The tincture or elixir strengths also make an excellent tea. I have also used chamomile combined with echinacea as a mouthwash in the treatment of canker sores.

New studies are also being conducted on the cancer-preventative activity of chamomile's active ingredient, apigenin. It seems that apigenin is showing promise as a sun blocker that is protective against ultraviolet light causing skin cancers. [13-15]

Dosage:

Take 350mg to 500mg in capsule form 3 to 4 times a day with food

Precautions:

Since chamomile is a member of the daisy family, anyone allergic to ragweed, asters or chrysanthemums should proceed with caution in using chamomile. [11,12] You may also want to keep in mind chamomile's tranquilizing effects if you are taking any other central nervous system depressants such as antihistamines. No contraindications have been shown for its use during pregnancy or lactation.

REFERENCES: CHAMOMILE

1.) Grieve, Mrs. M
   A Modern Herbal, pg. 185
   © 1931 Harcourt, Brace and Co, 1971 Dover Publication, NY, NY

2.) Hoffmann, David L
   The Herbalist
   Version 2.0 © 1992 CD-ROM Hopkins Technology, Hopkins, MN

3.) Tyler, Varro E
   Herbs of Choice: The Therapeutic Use of Phytomedicinals, pg. 57
   © 1994 Hawthorn Press Inc, Binghamton, New York 13904-1580

4.) Viola H, Wasowski C, Levi de Stein M, Wolfman C, Silveira R, Dajas F, Medina JH
Apigenin, a component of Matricaria recutita flowers is a central benzodiazepine receptors-ligand with anxiolytic effects
Planta Med 1995 Jun; 61 (3): 213-216

5.) Hoffmann, David L
The Herbalist
Version 2.0 © 1992 CD-ROM Hopkins Technology, Hopkins, MN

6.) Tyler, Varro E
Herbs of Choice: The Therapeutic Use of Phytomedicinals, pg. 58
© 1994 Hawthorn Press Inc, Binghamton, New York 13904-1580

7.) Tyler, Varro E
Herbs of Choice: The Therapeutic Use of Phytomedicinals, pg. 57
© 1994 Hawthorn Press Inc, Binghamton, New York 13904-1580

8.) Carle R and Isaac O
Zeitschrift fur Phytotherapie 8: 67-77 (1987)

9.) Mills, Simon Y
Out of the Earth: The Essential Book of Herbal Medicine, pg. 451
© 1991 Penguin Books, Viking Arkana, London

10.) Tierra, Lesley
The Herbs of life: Health and Healing using Western and Eastern Techniques, pg. 56
© 1992 The Crossing Press, Freedom, California 95019

11.) Brown, Donald J
Herbal Prescriptions for Better Health, pg. 55
© 1996 Prima Publishing, Rocklin, California 95677

12.) Mann C and Staba J
"The Chemistry, Pharmacology, and Commercial Formulations of Chamomile," in Herbs, Spices, and Medicinal Plants: Recent Advances in Botany, Horticulture, and Pharmacology
Vol. 1, LE Craker and JE Simon; eds
Oryx Press, Phoenix, Arizona 1986, pp. 233-280

Dandelion

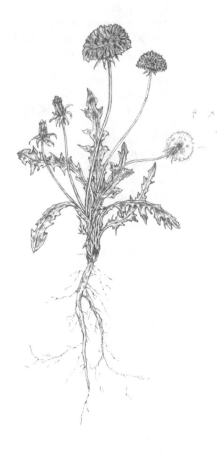

Dandelion (*Taraxacum officinale*). Just the mention of the name sends shivers down the spine of anyone trying to maintain an enviable "golf course" lawn. Everyone wants to get rid of it, but it is one of the best herbs that can be included in any list of phytotherapeutic medicinals.

The name "dandelion" is an Anglicized version of the French word *"dent-de-lion"* or "lion's tooth." It was given this name because of its jagged-edged leaves. The botanical name, *taraxacum*, is derived from the Greek *taraxos* which means disorder, and *akos*, which means remedy.[1] With this description, you can see why this lowly "weed" was used to treat a multitude of disorders. The root and leaves are used medicinally, although according to some, they produce different effects.

Mechanism of Action:

The main chemical ingredient of dandelion is taraxacin, a bitter resin, and taraxacerin, an acrid resin. Dandelion also contains phytosterols, gluten, gum and potash.[2] It also contains a very high concentration of potassium salts, 4.25 percent[3] and even contains a higher amount of Vitamin A than carrots (14,000 units vs. 11,000 units).[4-6] Besides Vitamin A, other active principles include iron, trace minerals, and Vitamins B and C.

Uses:

Dandelion has been used successfully as a diuretic and a remedy for the liver. A study that was conducted on animals has shown that dandelion is as effective as the prescription drug furosemide (Lasix®).[7] Because of its high content of potassium, dandelion leaf does not deplete the potassium that is stored in the cells, the way most non-potassium-sparing diuretics do. In this manner it replaces the lost potassium and achieves a more balanced effect. Some herbalists recommend that a stronger diuretic effect can be achieved if the leaves are used rather than the roots, which are recommended for their effects on the liver.

Dandelion root can also be used as an excellent liver tonic. This herb has been shown to improve the flow of bile from the liver by causing a direct increase in its production and a direct effect on the gall bladder by causing its contraction and release of stored bile.[8] It may therefore be helpful as an adjuvant therapy in the treatment of hepatitis, jaundice, and gall bladder inflammation (cholecystitis) provided that the bile ducts have not been blocked.

Dosage:

Capsules: 500mg to 1,000mg of the dry herb 3 to 4 times daily with food

Although some herbalists have used the leaves to achieve the diuretic effect and the roots for its effects on the liver, the recommended dosage still remains the same.

Since this herb does not concentrate well, it is not recommended that it be purchased in a tincture form. Tinctures contain alcohol and in order to achieve the recommended dosage, a high level of alcohol would need to be consumed.

Side Effects:

Although dandelion has been shown to be relatively free of side effects, a mild intestinal discomfort may occur which will dissipate with continued use. If this is a problem, take it with meals.

Cautions:

Because of dandelion's high potassium content, it should not be used on patients that are taking medications known as ACE inhibitors (Angiotensin Converting Enzyme), patients that have kidney problems, or diabetes mellitus. All of these can affect the absorption and excretion of potassium, which should be monitored closely with laboratory tests.

I would caution people not to pick wild dandelions from the side of the road. The plants may have been treated with pesticides and weed-killers. They may also have been exposed to large amounts of sodium or calcium chloride, especially if they are along the roadside. These chemicals are used to melt ice on the roadways, especially in colder climates.

REFERENCES: DANDELION

1.) Grieve, Mrs. M
   A Modern Herbal
   © 1931 and 1971 Dover Publications, Inc. 180 Barick St., NY, NY 10014 pg. 250

2.) Grieve, Mrs. M
   A Modern Herbal
   © 1931 Harcourt, Brace and Co, 1971 Dover Publication, New York, New York

3.) Mills, Simon Y.
   Out of the Earth: The Essential Book of Herbal Medicine
   © 1991 Penguin Books, Viking Arkana, London

4.) Murray, Michael T
   The Healing Power of Herbs
   © 1992 Prima Publishing, Rocklin, California 95677

5.) Leung AY: *Encyclopedia of Common Natural Ingredients Used in Food, Drugs and Cosmetics*
   John Wiley & Sons, NY, NY 1980

6.) Duke JA
   Handbook of Medicinal Herbs
   CRC Press, Boca Raton, Florida © 1985

7.) Raczkotilla E, et al
     The action of Taraxacum officianale extracts on the body weight and
     diuresis of laboratory animals
     Planta Medica 26, pg. 212-217, 1974

8.) Murray, Michael T
     The Healing Power of Herbs
     © 1992 Prima Publishing, Rocklin, California 95677

Echinacea

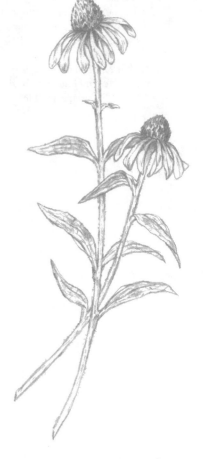

P urple cone flower, belonging to the sunflower family, *Echinachea purpurea* and *E. angustifolia*, are the two species most researched and most medically active. There are nine species of the plant that are native to North America and Canada. Two, unfortunately, have been placed on the endangered species list.

Mechanism of Action:

Echinacea has no direct bactericidal or bacteriostatic property.[1] It is a high molecular weight polysaccharide molecule, which is a non-specific immune stimulator. Polysaccharides are large sugar molecules that are distinctly different from other sugar molecules such as glucose and fructose (don't worry, you won't have to count your calories while taking these herbs). The majority of these effects appear to be caused by the binding of the active echinacea polysaccharides to carbohydrate receptors on the cell surface of macrophages and T-lymphocytes.[2] It therefore increases phagocytosis.

Phagocytosis can best be described as the human version of Pac-Man©. Another mechanism of action is echinacea's ability to inhibit the production of the enzyme hyaluronidase by certain pathogens that break down hyaluronic acid. Hyaluronic acid helps bind cells together.[3] This may be the reason Native

Americans knew of the healing properties of echinacea for the treatment of snakebites. Snake venom spreads through the body by its ability to breakdown hyaluronic acid. Echinacea is also found to increase interferon levels.[4,5]

Uses:

Echinacea can be used for the following:

• Prophylaxis and/or treatment of colds and flu-like symptoms of the upper respiratory tract such as laryngitis and tonsillitis

• Adult and pediatric otitis media (ear infections)

• Sinusitis

• Externally as an ointment for skin infections such as boils and carbuncles

• Adjuvant therapy for recurring vaginal *Candida albicans*.

• Lower urinary tract infections

• It may also be used as a gargle for sore throats[6-8]

One study has shown that echinacea may be useful in helping the immune system of patients with chronic fatigue syndrome (CFS) and acquired immunodeficiency syndrome.[9] Since both are considered autoimmune illnesses, echinacea, in these circumstances, should be used with caution.

Dosage and Administration:

There are many products of echinacea on the market. Some are also combined with other herbs so that a synergistic effect will take place. Echinacea works best if started at the very onset of a cold or flu. The recommended dose is dependent on the potency and form of the product used. In general, for acute situations, a dosage of 20 drops of the standardized tincture mixed in a little warm water (30 ml or about one ounce) or one capsule, may be taken every two hours for the first 48 hours, then 30 drops or one capsule every six hours for seven to 10 days or until symptoms subside. This should equal a daily dose of 900mg. For chronic use in supporting the immune system, 30 drops or one capsule every eight hours for three to four weeks with a one-week rest period. Pediatric doses can be calculated by following the recommended doses on the labeled product or may be calculated by using either Young's or Clark's Rule (see Appendix A).

Echinacea has been shown to be safe during pregnancy and lactation.

Caution:

Since echinacea is a non-specific immunostimulator, it should be used with caution in specific autoimmune illnesses such as:

- Lupus erythymatosis

- Tuberculosis

- Multiple sclerosis

This caution is based on speculation that stimulating an over-active immune system may be ill-advised. No controlled studies have been done to confirm the speculation.[10]

REFERENCES: ECHINACEA

1.) Tyler, Varro E
   Herbs of Choice: The Therapeutic Use of Phytomedicinals, pp. 182-184
   © 1994 Pharmaceutical Products Press, Binghamton, New York
   13904-1580

2.) Stimpel M, Proksch A, et al
   Macrophage activation and induction of macrophage cytotoxicity by
   purified polysaccharide fractions from the plant *Echinacea purpura*.
   Infect Immunity 46: 845-849, 1984

3.) Werbach, Melvin R and Murray, Michael T
   Botanical Influences on Illness, pg. 208
   © 1994 Third Line Press, Tarzana, California 91356

4.) Bauer R, Wagner H
   Echinacea species as potential immunostimulatory drugs
   Econ Med Res 5: 253-321, 1991

5.) Wacker A and Hilbig W
   Virus-inhibition by echinacea purpurea
   Plant Medica 33: 89-102, 1978

6.) Hobbs, Christopher
   Echinacea: A Literative Review
   Special supplement to *HerbalGram* # 30, 1994

7.) Foster, Steven
   Echinacea Education Monograph
   Quarterly Review of Natural Medicine, Winter Quarter, 1993 pp. 19-29

8.) Hoffmann, David L
   The Herbalist
   Version 2.0 © 1992 CD-ROM Hopkins Technology, Hopkins, MN

9.) See MD, Broumand N, Sahl L, Tilles JG
   In-vitro effects of echinacea and ginseng on natural killer and anti-body
   dependent cell cytotoxicity in healthy subjects and chronic fatigue
   syndrome or acquired immunodeficiency syndrome patients
   Immunopharmacology 1997, Jan; 35 (3): 229-235

10.)McCaleb, Rob
   Echinacea Safety Confirmed
   HerbalGram Number 42 Spring 1998

Evening Primrose Oil

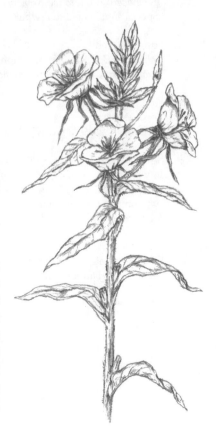

Evening primrose oil (EPO) contains a rich source of gamma-linoleic acid (GLA). GLA is also known as an essential fatty acid (EFA).

An essential fat? You don't usually see or hear those two words in the same sentence. As you may have guessed, some fats are needed for our bodies to function properly. This is very evident in infants where great amounts of EFAs and other fats are needed for proper cell growth and development.

Unfortunately, the American diet contains more of the unessential fats than the essential ones. Many people develop problems such as obesity, hypertension, and cardiac problems from an increase in fats that the body cannot utilize properly. Luckily, essential fatty acids are obtained from plant sources, not animal, thereby eliminating some of the detrimental fats such as cholesterol. (Cholesterol is only obtained from animal sources—not plants.)

Mechanism of Action:

Evening primrose oil is high in gamma linolenic acid (GLA), an essential fatty acid (EFA). Essential fatty acids can only be obtained through our diet; we cannot manufacture them.

In our bodies, EFAs undergo a series of complex reactions that convert the EFAs to substances, which can be utilized by the body.

Some people have problems with parts of this reaction, especially if they have difficulty utilizing the enzyme delta-6-desaturase. Delta-6-desaturase helps start the beginning part of the reactions that transform EFAs to a form which can be used by our bodies so they may be more easily converted to prostaglandins. Prostaglandins help regulate many of the metabolic functions that occur in our bodies.

Other sources that could hinder the utilization of EFAs are viruses, alcohol, insufficient zinc or insulin, excessive trans-fatty acid intake, and the aging process.

(Also see the Evening Primrose Oil information under Gynecological Disorders in Part One.)

Feverfew

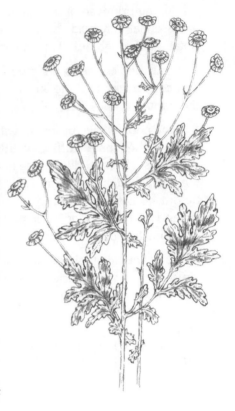

Feverfew (*Tanacetum parthenium*) has been used as an anti-pyretic (a drug that reduces fever) since the first century AD. It is native to Europe and the United States and is a member of the daisy family. The leaves are used for medicinal purposes. It is also known as midsummer daisy, featherfew and featherfoil.[1]

Mechanism of Action:

Feverfew contains chemical compounds called sesquiterpene lactones (STLs). The most important of these is called parthenolide. Parthenolide is responsible for most of feverfew's medicinal actions. The concentration of parthenolide can vary greatly depending upon where the plants were harvested and also what time of year they were harvested. Parthenolide seems to exert its effect by inhibiting the release of blood vessel dilating substances (seratonin and histamine) from platelets, inhibiting the production of inflammatory substances (leukotrienes, serine proteases, etc.), and re-establishing proper blood vessel tone.[2,3] It can be classified as an herbal anti-prostaglandin. (Prostaglandins are natural substances in the body that cause either constriction or dilation of blood vessels and vascular areas.)

Uses:

- Migraine Headaches
- Inflammation
- Rheumatoid Arthritis

Feverfew has been used successfully for the prevention and treatment of migraine headaches. Migraines have either been eliminated, the severity of the attacks have been lessened, or the length of time between attacks had been increased.

The efficacy of feverfew is dependent upon adequate levels of parthenolide, the active ingredient. The preparations used in successful clinical trials have a parthenolide content of 0.4 to 0.66 percent.[4-6] This equates to a low dosage of approximately 400 micrograms (mcg) of parthenolide. Standardization must be adhered to with the use of this herb.

Dosage:

A standardized preparation of at least 0.4 percent or higher of parthenolide content should be taken daily. This is equivalent to approximately 400 micrograms of the active ingredient. The daily amount of the drug should be in the range of 25mg to 75mg two times daily. Some formulations can be taken once daily. Feverfew works best if taken at bedtime. This will ensure enough of the active ingredient will be in the blood stream during the early morning hours when most migraines occur. It may take anywhere between one to two months to see an improvement. During an acute attack, the dosage of feverfew may be increased to one tablet three to four times daily. As an anti-inflammatory, the dosage range would be a standardized dosage (400 to 600 mcg) taken three to four times daily.

Cautions:

Feverfew should **NOT** be used during pregnancy or lactation. It should also not be used if the patient is also taking any type of anti-coagulant therapy.

Some people have been known to chew on the fresh leaves. This has produced mouth ulcers in sensitive individuals.

REFERENCES: FEVERFEW

1.) Hoffmann, David L
The Herbalist
Version 2.0 © 1992 CD-ROM Hopkins Technology, Hopkins, MN

2.) Awang DVC
Feverfew
Can Pharm J 122: 266-270, 1989

3.) Werbach, Melvin R and Murray, Michael T
Botanical Influences on Illness pg. 171
© 1994 Third Line Press, Tarzana, California 91356

4.) Werbach, Melvin R and Murray, Michael T
Botanical Influences on Illness pg. 172
© 1994 Third Line Press, Tarzana, California 91356

5.) Heptinstall S, et al
Parthenolide content and bioactivity of feverfew (Tanacetum parthenium (L.) Schultz-Bip) Estimation of commercial and authenti-cated feverfew products
J Pharm Pharmacol 44: 391-395, 1992

6.) Brown AM, Edwards CM, Davey MR, Power JB, Lowe KC
Pharmacological activity of feverfew (Tanacetum parthenium (L.) Schultz-Bip): assessment by inhibition of human polymorphonuclear leukocyte chemiluminescence in-vitro
J Pharm Pharmacol 1997 May; 49 (5): 558-561

Garlic

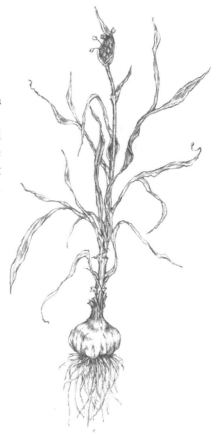

G arlic, *Allium sativum*, is a member of the lily family. It has been used as both food and medicine dating back to the Egyptian Pharaohs and ancient China. Garlic is even mentioned in the Bible's Old Testament.[1]

Mechanism of Action:

Garlic undergoes a series of reactions in order for its medicinal properties to be achieved. It contains the odorless and sulfur-containing amino acid, alliin. When garlic is crushed or chewed, the alliin comes in contact with other cells containing the enzyme alliinase. Alliinase converts alliin to allicin. Allicin is the sulfur-containing compound that has many of the medicinal properties.

Alliin—> Allinase enzyme—> Allicin (medicinally active)

Allicin is not a very stable compound. The acid environment of the stomach inactivates it. Garlic tablets should therefore be enteric-coated in order to prevent the breakdown of the allicin in the stomach and dissolve in a less hostile alkaline environment of the small intestine.[2,3]

Uses:

Although garlic has a wide range of well-documented effects, its most important clinical effects are anti-microbial and cardiovascular.[4]

111

Antimicrobial

Garlic has been shown to inhibit the growth of the following organisms:

- *Staphylococcus aureus*
- *E. coli*
- *Bacillus cereus*
- *Mycobacterium smegmatis*
- *Klebsiella pneumoniae* [5]

Antifungal

Garlic has been shown to inhibit the growth of many fungi such as *Microsporum, Trichophyton* and *Aspergillus.*[6-7] It has been shown to be effective against fungi that affect the skin. Concentrated garlic oil applied to infected areas of the skin, especially around the ears, fingers and toes, has been shown to produce effective results and has been shown to be active against Candida albicans.[8]

Cardiovascular

This is where garlic can be used to its greatest advantage. Studies have shown that garlic interferes with the production of cholesterol in the liver and also increases the level of serum high-density lipoproteins (HDL—the good cholesterol).[9,10]

One study showed that at a daily dose of 900mg, LDL-cholesterol and triglycerides were reduced by 21 percent and 24 percent respectively.[11] Garlic has also been shown to decrease blood pressure by as much as 20 to 30mmHg for the systolic pressure (top number) and 10 to 20mmHg for the diastolic pressure (bottom number).[12,13]

Diabetes Mellitus

Another study has shown that garlic may be helpful in the treatment of diabetes mellitus by showing a hypoglycemic effect. This is caused by garlic's increasing the metabolism of glucose.[14] Garlic's active ingredient, allicin, competes with insulin for insulin-inactivating sites in the liver. If the sites are bound, then insulin cannot be destroyed. This results in more free insulin circulating in the blood stream to help metabolize glucose.

Dosage:

The dosing of garlic should be based on the allicin content of the preparation. Therapeutic effects are seen when the daily allicin ingestion is 3,000 to 5,000mcg in divided doses.

Since allicin is sensitive to high acidity, the enteric-coated form is best, so take it on an empty stomach. This will ensure that the tablet is dissolved in the small intestine and not in the low acid pH environment of the stomach. Avoid the use of oral oil capsules, since the oil may become rancid and lose any medicinal properties over time.

Caution:

Garlic has been shown to increase the clotting time in some individuals, therefore caution should be used on patients taking anti-coagulant medication (e.g., Coumadin®).

Since allicin is a sulfur-containing compound, caution should be exercised in persons with a hypersensitivity to sulfur, although this reaction is very rare.

Side effects:

Excessive garlic intake has been shown to produce minor gastro-intestinal disturbances and flatulence (gas).

REFERENCES: GARLIC

1.) Old Testament Book of Numbers II
    Good News Bible
    © 1976 American Bible Society

2.) Tyler, Varro E.
    Herbs of choice: The Therapeutic Use of Phytomedicinals
    © 1994 Hawthorn Press Inc., Binghamton, New York 13904-1580

3.) Brown, Donald J
   Herbal Prescriptions for Better Health
   © 1996 Prima Publishing, Rocklin, California 95677

4.) Murray, Michael
   The Healing Power of Herbs
   © 1992 Prima Publishing, Rocklin, California 95677

5.) Naganawa R, Iwata N, Ishikawa K, Fukuda H, Fujino T, Suzuki A
   Inhibition of microbial growth by ajoene, a sulfur-containing compound derived from garlic
   Appl Environ Microbiol 1996 Nov; 62 (11) 4238-4242

6.) Amer M, Taha and Tosson Z
   The effect of aqueous garlic extraction on the growth of dermatophytes
   Int. J Dermatol 1980 19:285-287

7.) Pai ST, Platt MW
   Antifungal effects of Allium sativum (garlic) extract against the Aspergillus species involved in otomycosis
   Lett Appl Microbiol 1995 Jan; 20 (1):14-18

8.) Moore GS, Atkins RD
   The fungicidal and fungistatic effects of an aqueous garlic extract on medically important yeast-like fungi
   Mycologia 69: 341-348 1977

9.) Efendy JL, Simmons DL, Campbell GR, Campbell JH
   The effect of the aged garlic extract, Kyolic, on the development of experimental atherosclerosis
   Atherosclerosis 1997 Jul 11; 132 (1): 37-42

10.) Orekhov AN, Grunwald J
   Effects of garlic on atherosclerosis
   Nutrition 1997 Jul; 13 (7-8): 656-663

11.) Holzgartner H, Schmidt U, Kuhn U
   Comparison of the efficacy and tolerance of a garlic preparation vs. bezafibrate
   Arzneim-Forsch Drug Res 42: pg. 1473-1477 1992

12.) Foushee DB, Ruffin J, Banerjee U
   Garlic as a natural agent for the treatment of hypertension a preliminary report
   Cytobios 34: 145-62 1982

13.) Murray, Michael
   The Healing Power of Herbs
   © 1992 Prima Publishing, Rocklin, California 95677

14.) Bever BO, Zahnd GR
   Plants with oral hypoglycemic action
   Quart J Crude Drug Res 1979: 17: 139-96

Ginger

Although thought of as a root, ginger is actually a rhizome (an underground stem) from the plant *Zingiber officinale*. Ginger is grown in many parts of the world and is distinguished by its name (Chinese ginger, Jamaican ginger, etc.). Ginger has been used for centuries as both a flavoring agent and a medicinal agent[1]

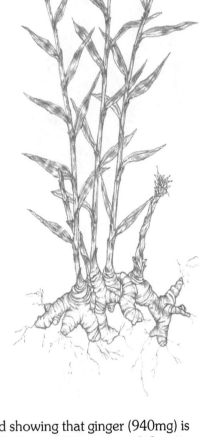

Mechanism of Action:

The plant contains numerous volatile oils of which zingiberene and bisabolene are the most active. Other oils are also responsible for ginger's odor, taste, and activity (gingerols and shogaols).

Uses:

• Anti-nauseant

• Anti-emetic (deters vomiting)

Studies have been conducted showing that ginger (940mg) is as effective as 100mg of dimenhydrinate (Dramamine®)[2] in the control of nausea and vomiting especially when associated with motion sickness. Ginger seems to work on the gastro-intestinal tract by slowing down the feedback mechanism from the brain to the CTZ (Chemo-receptor Trigger Zone) and not on the central nervous system thus eliminating many of the side effects associated with central nervous system-type anti-nauseants (which produce dry mouth, blurry vision and sedation).

Dosage:

Ginger may be given in the form of 500mg capsules. It is recommended that 1000 mg be given one hour prior to departure for controlling symptoms of motion sickness and continue taking one to two capsules (500mg to 1000mg) every four to six hours.

Cautions:

The German Commission E suggests that ginger should not be used by persons with gall stones.[3] Ginger has been shown to affect platelet aggregation and clotting time with patients on anticoagulant therapy, but this usually happens when higher doses are given (10gm).[4] Patients should be questioned routinely about their intake of certain herbs (especially ginger), if they are having surgery since they could affect the results of post-operative recovery.[5]

Ginger has been used for *hyperemesis gravidarum* (severe nausea and vomiting during pregnancy). This should only be conducted under the close supervision of a trained clinician.[6]

Other Suggested Uses:

• German Commission E has also approved the use of ginger in the treatment of dyspepsia (indigestion).

• Ginger may show promise as an effective anti-emetic (anti-vomiting) for same-day surgery cases[7] and may also be used as a pre-treatment anti-nauseant and anti-emetic before chemotherapy.[8]

• Ginger was also found to exert anti-inflammatory properties.[9] Therefore, *one* drug could be used in minor surgical procedures as an anti-inflammatory and an anti-emetic. Managed care should love that!

REFERENCES: GINGER

1.) Hoffmann, David L
The Herbalist
Version 2.0 © 1992 CD-ROM Hopkins Technology, Hopkins, MN

2.) Mowrey DB, Clayson DE
Motion sickness, ginger, and psychophysics
Lancet I; 655-657, 1982

3.) Monograph, Zingiberis rhizomo Bundesanzeiger 5/5/88 (German Commission E)

4.) Bordia A, Vorma SK, Srivastava KC
Effect of ginger (Zingiber officinale Rosc) and fenugreek (Trigonella foenumgraecum L) on blood lipids, blood sugar and platelet aggregation in patients with coronary artery disease
Prostaglandins-Leukot-Essent-Fatty-Acids © 1997 May; 56 (5): 379-384

5.) Backon J
Ginger as an antiemetic: possible side effects due to its thromboxane synthetase activity
Letter Anaesthesia 46 (8): 669-671, 1991

6.) Fischer-Rasmussen W, Kjaer SK, et al
Ginger treatment of hyperemesisgravidarum
Eur J Obstet Gynecol Reprod Biol 38; 19-24, 1980

7.) Philips S, Ruggier R, Hutchinson SE
Zingiber officinale (ginger)—an antiemetic for day case surgery
Anaesthesia 1993 Aug; 48 (8): 715-717

8.) Sharma SS, Kochupillai V, Gupta SK, Seth SD, Gupta YK
Antiemetic efficacy of ginger (Zingiber officinale) against cisplatin-induced emesis in dogs
J Ethnopharmacol 1997 Jul 57 (2): 93-96

9.) Srivatava KC, Mustafa T
Ginger (Zingiber officinale) in rheumatism and musculoskeletal disorders
Med-Hypotheses 1992 Dec; 39 (4): 342-348

Ginkgo Biloba

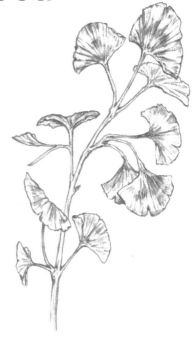

G inkgo biloba, sometimes called the "maiden hair tree," is the oldest living species of tree that is known today. Fossils have been found which show that it has been in existence for over 200 million years! The ginkgo tree has shown tremendous resistance to insects, disease and the pollution of modern life.

Ginkgo leaf extracts are now among the leading herbal medicines in both Germany and France. The extracts account for 1.0 percent and 1.5 percent of total prescription sales in Germany and France, respectively. Over 100,000 physicians worldwide combined to write more than 10,000,000 prescriptions in 1989.[1] The leaves are used medicinally, although in Chinese medicine, the seeds are also used. We will restrict our discussions here to the use of the leaves.

Mechanism of Action:

Ginkgo biloba contains a complex array of medicinally active ingredients. Again, Mother Nature is up to her old synergistic tricks where an isolated component never works as well as when they are all together. Extract of ginkgo biloba, (or EGb), is standardized to 24 percent ginkgo flavone glycosides and 6 percent terpene lactones. The flavonoid glycosides are mainly quercetin and kaempferol. The terpene molecules are the ginkgolides

A, B and C and the sesquiterpene bilobalide. These compounds are only contained in ginkgo biloba and not in any other plants.[2-4] The plant has extremely powerful anti-oxidant properties and free radical scavenger effects. When all of this is taken collectively, EGb exerts its effect by increasing the blood flow to the brain and extremities, therefore increasing the amount of oxygen available to the organs. This would also pave the way for better use of blood glucose and an increase in energy.

Uses:

The venerable ginkgo biloba comes with a long list of extensive uses. A short list would include:

- Alzheimer's disease
- Asthma
- Circulatory problems
- Depression
- Impaired memory
- Improved nerve cell functioning and message transmission
- Intermittent claudication
- Platelet-activating factor (PAF) antagonism
- Raynaud's disease
- Stroke complications
- Tinnitis
- Vascular disorders
- Vertigo

I think you can see why ginkgo is so widely used. To simplify things, I've grouped the effects into four distinctive categories.

1. Cerebral insufficiencies
2. Tinnitis and vertigo

3. Peripheral vascular disorders

4. Ophthalmic disorders

Let's take a look at some of the more clinically documented tests.

Cerebral Insufficiencies

The challenges of "just getting old" are many. Cerebral vascular insufficiency, or CVI, can be classified as a lack of oxygen to the brain. Memory loss, depression, lack of concentration and disorientation are just some of the problems consistent with CVI and what the aging baby-boomer generation is facing. EGb increases the cerebral blood flow to the brain. This in turn supplies the brain with energy in the form of more oxygen and glucose. EGb also inhibits platelet-activating factor (PAF). When PAF is released by the cells, it causes platelet aggregation (clumping), arterial thrombosis (clotting), acute inflammation, allergic reactions and a variety of cardiovascular effects.[5] Studies have been conducted with EGb using sophisticated measurements of assessment (Crichton's, Stockton's, Sandoz Clinical Assessment Geriatric Scale (SCAG) and Folstein Mini-mental State Exam, just to name a few). In one study showing the efficacy of EGb in the treatment of mild to moderate primary degenerative dementia of the Alzheimer type, 216 patients were placed on either a placebo or 120mg twice daily of standardized EGb. Of these, 156 patients completed the 24-week study. There was a significant improvement in the EGb group over the placebo group.[6] They had less depression and dementia and their cognitive functions improved.

In another study, 309 patients were assessed over a 52-week period on a dose of 40mg three times a day. The results showed that ginkgo improved the cognitive performance and social functioning of demented patients for six months to one year.[7]

Many other tests have been performed on the use of EGb in the treatment of Alzheimer's disease. More work needs to be done, but it seems that EGb does seem to slow the progression of this extremely debilitating disease.

The term "resistant depression" which can be used to describe depression that is unresponsive to prescriptions and/or herbal antidepressants has been shown to be controlled with EGb. In one study, assessment of depression on the Hamilton Depression Scale was cut in half, from 14 to 7.[8]

In the treatment of depression in the elderly, cerebral insufficiency should be the first thought that comes to our minds. Unfortunately, we usually put patients on an antidepressant with its own set of side effects, without really getting to the heart of the matter which is the lowered amount of oxygen to the brain.[9] Not only should EGb be used, but also an increase in activity, both mental and especially physical (any type of exercise or physical movement), should be incorporated in the treatment regimen.

Tinnitis and Vertigo

The causes of tinnitis (ringing in the ears) and vertigo (a sensation that has been described as if everything around you is spinning), can be very difficult to determine. Many people, especially senior citizens, can be susceptible to the problems of the organs of the inner ear caused by anoxia (a lack of oxygen) often times due to atherosclerosis (a hardening of the arteries). In blind and double blind studies, ginkgo was shown to be superior to a placebo in 40 to 80 percent of the patients in the test groups. The tests were conducted on patients who showed symptoms of acute or chronic dizziness with or without tinnitis, and in those patients who experienced vertigo who had definite inner ear disturbances caused by trauma, Meniere's disease or infection.[10-14] All the results were positive and pointed to ginkgo's effectiveness in the management of hearing and equilibrium disturbances.

Peripheral Vascular Disorders

Intermittent claudication is best described as cramping and pain in the lower legs (especially the calf) when walking. It is due primarily to poor peripheral circulation in the veins. EGb has been shown to be effective in this disorder.[15] It has also been shown to be effective in other circulatory disorders such as Raynaud's disease (cold hands and feet).[16]

Ophthalmic Disorders

Diabetics, especially elderly diabetics, whether on insulin or not, are much more susceptible to the degeneration of the arteries and veins that carry blood to the eyes. When these tiny capillaries become blocked, senile macular degeneration or retinal insufficiency can develop. At the end of one study,[17] visual acuity (how clearly we see) and visual field (how much we see) as measured by funduscopic examination had improved by almost four times (2.3 diopters) over the placebo group (0.6 diopters).

Dosage:

EGb's (extract ginkgo biloba) beneficial effects can usually be seen if it is taken consistently for at least four to six months. The recommended daily dosage is 120 to 240mg in divided doses of either two to three times daily (40mg to 80mg) with meals, using the standardized 24 percent extract. The 240mg is usually reserved for cerebral insufficiencies. Because so much of the plant is used to achieve a 24 percent extract, the beneficial effects of ginkgo cannot be achieved by drinking a tea.[18]

Cautions and Side effects:

Due to its PAF (platelet-activating factor) effects, EGb should be used with caution in patients receiving anti-coagulant therapy. This would include both warfarin compounds and aspirin. Do *not* use if pregnant. Some people have also experienced mild gastrointestinal problems.[19]

REFERENCES: GINKGO BILOBA

1.) Werbach, Melvin R and Murray, Michael T
Botanical Influences on Illness
© 1994 Third Line Press, Tarzana, California 91356

2.) Murray, Michael T
The Healing Power of Herbs, pp. 118-132

© 1992 Prima Publishing, Rocklin, California 95677

3.) Tyler, Varro E
   Herbs of Choice: The Therapeutic Use of Phytomedicinals pp.108-111
   © 1994 Hawthorn Press Inc, Binghamton, New York 13904-1580

4.) Crisp P, O'Brien J, McTavish D
   Ginkgo biloba Extract (Egb761) in perspective
   Science Press, Hong Kong © 1993
   Adis International Ltd, New Zealand

5.) Kroegel C
   The potential pathophysiological role of platelet activating factor in
   human diseases
   Klinische Wochenschrift 66: 373-378, 1988

6.) Kanowski S, Herrman WM, et al
   Efficacy and tolerability of the Ginkgo biloba extract EGb 761 in
   outpatients with presinile and senile Alzheimer-type dementia and
   multi-infarct dementia
   Abstract from the Sixth Congress of the International Psychogeriatric
   Association, Berlin, Sept 5-10, 1993

7.) LeBars Ph, Katz MM, Berman N, Iutil TM, Freedman AM, Schatzberg AF
   A Placebo-controlled, Double-blind, Randomized Trial of an Extract of
   Ginkgo Biloba for Dementia
   JAMA 1997; 278: 1327-1332

8.) Lesser IM, Mena I, et al
   Reduction in cerebral blood flow in older depressed patients
   Arch Gen Psychiatr 51: 677-686 1994

9.) Brown, Donald J
   Herbal Prescriptions for Better Health, pp. 119-128
   © 1996 Prima Publishing, Rocklin, California 95677

10.) Claussen E, Claussen CF
   Comparative study on the treatment of dizziness and tinnitus with
   Rokan®
   *Proceedings dem Gesellschaft Fur Neurootologic und
   Aequilibriometrie*, Vol 7, pp. 471-485, 1981

11.) Haquenaner JP, Cantenot F, Koskas H, Pierart H
   Treatment of disturbed equilibrium with Ginkgo biloba extract-
   multicenter double-blind study versus placebo
   Press Medicale 15: 1569-1572, 1986

12.) Hamann K-F
Physical treatment of vestibular vertigo in relation to Ginkgo biloba extract
Therapiewoche 35: 4586-4590, 1985

13.) Meyer B
A multicenter randomized double-blind study of Ginkgo biloba extract versus placebo in the treatment of tinnitus
Press Medicale 15: 1562-1564, 1986

14.) Schwerdtfeger F
Electronystagmographically and clinically documented therapy with Rokan ® in the symptoms of dizziness
Therapiewoche 31: 8658-8667, 1981

15.) Bauer U
Ginkgo biloba extract in the treatment of arteriopathy of the lower limbs. Sixty-five week study
In Funfgeld EW (Ed) Rokan (Ginkgo biloba). Recent results in pharmacology and clinic, pp 212-220, Springer-Verlag, Berlin, Heidelberg, New York 1988

16.) Frileux C, Cope R
The concentrated extract of Ginkgo biloba in peripheral vascular disease
Cahiers d'Arteriologie de Royat 3: 117-122, 1975

17.) Lebuisson DA, Leroy L, Rigal G
Treatment of senile macular degeneration with Ginkgo biloba extract-a preliminary double-blind study versus placebo
Press Medicale 15: 1556-1558, 1986

18.) Tyler, Varro E
Herbs of Choice: The Therapeutic Use of Phytomedicinals, pp. 108-111
© 1994 Hawthorn Press Inc, Binghamton, New York 13904-1580

19.) Stalleiken D, Ihm P
Continuous observation of cognitive deficits. Results of a mulitcentre study conducted on the basis of psychological tests.
Therapiewoche (Suppl 2): 1-8, 1988

Ginseng
(Siberian and Chinese/Korean)

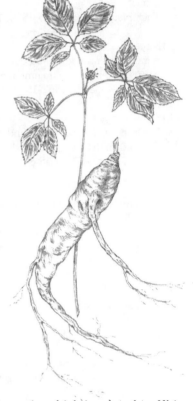

S ince there are more similarities in their actions than differences, *Panax ginseng*, C.E. Meyer (also known as either Chinese or Korean ginseng), and Siberian ginseng (*Eleutherococcus senticosus*) will be discussed together. The differences lie within their chemical structures. The root of both plants is used for its medicinal properties.

Mechanism of Action:

Eleutherococcus senticosus (Siberian ginseng), also known as eleuthero, is a distant cousin which is related to Chinese or Korean ginseng (*Panax*). Although not as well known as the more popular *Panax*, eleuthero's popularity as a medicinal herb dates back 2,000 years in the annals of Chinese medicine and dates back a few hundred years to its use by the people of Siberia (hence the name). Eleuthero is a thorny shrub, which grows anywhere between five to ten feet tall and is most abundant in the Far East, Korea, China and Japan. Eleuthero's activity is based on its content of eleutherosides, seven of which have been identified.[1]

Eleutherosides should not be confused with ginsenosides, which are the active ingredients of *Panax ginseng*. *Panax ginseng* C.E. Meyer, is probably the best known of the ginseng family. There are also other species of *Panax* such as *P.*

quinquefolius (American ginseng), *P. trifolium, P. japonicum,* C.E. Meyer (Japanese ginseng) and *P. pseudoginseng* (Himalayan ginseng).

Panax ginseng's active constituents are called ginsenosides or panaxosides.[2]

They total 13 and are identified by the letter R with a subscript letter or letter and number (i.e. Rb_1, Re, Rg_2).[3] The *Panax* species are identified by the existence or absence of the ginsenosides.

Remember:

Ginsenosides are not exactly eleutherosides and vice versa. Ginsenosides are all saponin glycosides. Eleutherosides contain both saponins and terpene compounds. As they say, the same but different.

Uses:

According to Russian pharmacologists I.I. Brekhman and I.V. Dardyma, ginsengs fall into a category called "adaptogens." By their definition, an adaptogen is any substance that:

1. Has a normalizing or balancing action that is independent of the direction of the pathological state.

2. Is harmless and will not cause disruption of normal physiological actions.

3. Has a non-specific action.[3-6]

By this definition, the ginsengs help the body normalize or balance the functions of a number of systems of the body (CNS, endocrine, etc.). In Oriental medicine, this would be defined as a balance between "yin and yang."

Both Panax and eleuthro ginsengs may be used for the following conditions:

Anti-fatigue (mental and physical) and Anti-stress

The ginsengs indirectly stimulate adrenal function by affecting the pituitary-adrenal feedback mechanism. With the adrenals producing more ACTH and functioning more efficiently, stress and fatigue are reduced and mental clarity is increased.[7]

Panax ginseng has also been shown to stimulate the immune function of chronic-fatigue syndrome patients and patients with acquired-immune deficiency syndrome.[8]

Increased Physical Ability

The ginsengs improve athletic ability by increasing the uptake of oxygen by the body for better utilization by the muscles. The ginsengs have also been shown to shorten recovery time after a strenuous workout.[9,10]

Helps Lower Cholesterol

The ginsengs help the liver metabolize cholesterol in a more efficient manner.[11] Ginseng also reduces platelet aggregation (stickiness).

Increases Immune System Function

Studies have shown that the ginsengs increase the production of lymphocytes and phagocytosis[12] which help the body increase its resistance to invading organisms.

Miscellaneous

The ginsengs may also help reduce the blood sugar of non-insulin dependent diabetics (Type 2).[13] Some success has also been achieved in using the ginsengs during menopause.[14,15] (Also see section on Menopause.)

Cautions:

The ginsengs may increase clotting time for patients taking warfarin therapy. Over-consumption has been associated with what has been called "ginseng-abuse syndrome." This was reported in the *Journal of the American Medical Association.* The article states that increased blood pressure, excessive CNS stimulation, nausea, diarrhea, and insomnia were reported.[16] But these findings were in only 10 percent of the patients surveyed, all of whom were drinking large amounts of coffee. In fact, all of the symptoms that were observed are consistent with caffeine addiction! Ginseng should be used with caution with people who take excessive amounts of caffeine-containing products. It is advisable that ginseng *not* be used during pregnancy or lactation.

Dosage:

Dosage for either the Panax or Siberian: 100mg to 500mg 3 times a day with food.

Standardization is the key word when recommending any form of ginseng be it Panax or Eleuthro. Adulterated products are plentiful especially for the Panax variety. This is one herb where the buyer should be aware of what he or she is purchasing. Whichever one is chosen, it is suggested to use the recommended dose of the product for about four to six weeks, discontinue its use for two weeks, then resume therapy. This will help the body adjust to a natural balance.

REFERENCES: GINSENG

1.) Farnsworth NR, Kinghorn AD, Soejarto DD, Waller DP
Siberian ginseng (*Eleutherococcus senticosus*): Current status as an adaptogen.
In: Economic and Medicinal Plant Research, Vol. 1
Academic Press, London 1985, pp. 155-215

2.) Tyler, Varro E
Herbs of Choice: The Therapeutic Use of Phytomedicinals, pg. 172
© 1994 Hawthorn Press Inc, Binghamton, New York 13904-1580

3.) Shibata S, Tanaka O, et al
Chemistry and pharmacology of *Panax*
In: Economic and Medicinal Plant Research, Vol. 1
Academic Press, London, 1985 pp. 217-284

4.) Murray, Michael T
The Healing Power of Herbs, pg. 41

5.) Brekhman II, Dardymov IV,
New substances of plant origin which increase nonspecific resistance
Ann Rev Pharmacol 9: 419-430, 1969

6.) Brekhman II, Dardymov IV
Pharmacological investigation of glycosides from ginseng and
Eleutherococcus Lloydia 32: 46-51, 1969

7.) Filaretou AA, Bogdanova TS, Podviginia, Bodganov AI
Role of Pituitary-adrenalcortical system in body adaptation abilities
Exp Clin Endocrinol 1988 Dec; 92 (2) 129-136

8.) See DM, Broumand N, Sahl, L, Tilles JG
In vitro effects of echinacea and ginseng on natural killer and anti-
body-dependent cell cytotoxicity in healthy subjects and chronic fatigue
syndrome or acquired immunodeficiency syndrome patients
Immunopharmacology 1997 Jan; 35 (3): 229-235

9.) Banerjee U, Izquierdo JA
Anti-stress and anti-fatigue properties of Panax ginseng: comparison
with piracetam
Acta Physiol Lat AM 1982; 32 (4): 277-285

10.) Pieralisi G, Ripari P, Vecchiet L
Effects of a standardized ginseng extract combined with
dimethylaminoethanol bitartrate, vitamins, minerals, and trace
elements on physical performance during exercise
Clin Ther 1991 May; 13 (3): 373-382

11.) Yamamoto M, Uemura T, et al
Serum HDL-cholesterol-increasing and fatty liver-improving actions of
Panax ginseng in high cholesterol diet-fed rats with clinical effect on
hyperlipidemia in man
Am J Chin Med 11: 1-4, 1983

12.) Bohn B, Nebe CT, Birr C
Flow-cytometric studies with *Eleutherococcus senticosus* extract as an
immunomodulating agent
Arzneim-Forsch Drug Res 37: 1193-1196, 1987

13.) Sotaniemi EA, Haapakoski E, Rautio A
Ginseng therapy in non-insulin-dependent diabetic patients
Diabetes Care 1995, Oct: 18 (10): 1373-1375

14.) Punnonen R, Lukola A
Oestrogen-like effect of ginseng
Br Med J 1980 Oct 25; 281 (6248): 1110

15.) Duda RB, Taback B, Kessel B, Dooley DD, Yang H, Marchiori J,
Slomovic BM, Alvarez JG
pS2 expression induced by American ginseng in MCF-7 breast cancer cells
Amn Surg Ocnol 1996 Nov; 3 (6): 515-520

16.) Siegel RK
Ginseng Abuse syndrome
JAMA 241: 1641-1615, 1979

Goldenseal

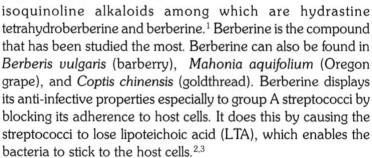

Goldenseal (*Hydrastis canadensis L.*), also known as yellow root, is a small perennial plant that grows in the damp ground of eastern North America. The root and rhizomes are the medically active part of the plant.

Mechanism of Action:

Since goldenseal is a plant native to North America, the early settlers of this country learned about the value of this herb from our Native American fathers. Goldenseal contains numerous isoquinoline alkaloids among which are hydrastine tetrahydroberberine and berberine.[1] Berberine is the compound that has been studied the most. Berberine can also be found in *Berberis vulgaris* (barberry), *Mahonia aquifolium* (Oregon grape), and *Coptis chinensis* (goldthread). Berberine displays its anti-infective properties especially to group A streptococci by blocking its adherence to host cells. It does this by causing the streptococci to lose lipoteichoic acid (LTA), which enables the bacteria to stick to the host cells.[2,3]

Uses:

Anti-infective

Goldenseal shows great promise with a broad range of antibiotic effects especially against group A streptococci bacteria. Since the berberine alkaloids show an affinity for other bacteria and fungi,[4-6] goldenseal would be an ideal adjuvant in the treatment of any inflammation involving the mucous membranes. Recent studies on different analogs of berberine have shown them to be effective against *Staphylococcus aureus.*[7]

Anti-diarrheal

Goldenseal has been used for the treatment of diarrhea caused by the following organisms: *E.coli, Shigella dysenteriae, Salmonella and Giardia lamblia.*[8-10]

A suggestion to travelers going to countries of questionable food and water quality would be to start taking goldenseal at home.

Dosage:

A standardized extract of between 5 to 15 percent of berberine should be used. This would be in the range of 250 to 500mg. There are products that combine goldenseal with other anti-infectives such as echinacea. The dose should be taken four times daily. A dose of *Lactobacillus acidophilus* should also be given with goldenseal because of its antibacterial properties. Acidophilus and other beneficial bacteria (*bifidobacterium*) which inhabit the gastro-intestinal tract should be given every time any anti-infective is given whether it is of herbal or prescription origin. This will prevent any over growth of fungal infections that may occur in any of the mucous membranes.

Cautions:

Berberine-containing plants should not be taken during pregnancy or lactation. They should also be supplemented with doses of B vitamins since berberine may interfere with their metabolism.[11] Unlike echinacea, goldenseal should not be used for long periods of time for immune-stimulating effects. Goldenseal should also be used with caution in diabetics since it may produce a hypoglycemic effect (lowering of the blood sugar).

REFERENCES: GOLDENSEAL

1.) Agricultural Research Service
Phytochemical and Ethnobotanical Databases USDA-ARS-NGRL
Stephen M Beckstrom-Sternberg and James A Duke
www.ars-grin.gov/~ngrlsb/index.html

2.) Werbach, Melvin R and Murray, Michael T
Botanical Influences of Illness
© 1994 Third Line Press, Tarzana, California 91356

3.) Sun D, Courtney HS, Beachey EH
Berberine sulfate blocks adherence of Streptococcus pyogenes to
epithelial cells, fibronectin and hexadecane
Antimicrob Agents Chemother 32: 1370-1374, 1988

4.) Hahn FE, Ciak J
Berberine
Antibiotics 3: 577-588, 1976

5.) Amin AH, Subbiah TV, Abbasi KM
Berberine Sulfate: Antimicrobial activity, bioassay, and mode of action
Can J Microbiology 15: 1067-1076, 1969

6.) Murray, Michael T
The Healing Power of Herbs
© 1992 Prima Publishing, Rocklin, California 95677

7.) Iwasa K, Kamigauchi M, Sugiura M, Nanba H
Antimicrobial activity of some 13-alkyl substituted protoberberinium salts
Planta Med 1997 Jun; 63 (3): 196-198

8.) Gupta S
Use of berberine in the treatment of giardiasis
Am J Dis Child 129: 866, 1975

9.) Bhakat MP, Nandi N, Pal HK, Khan BS
Therapeutic trial of berberine sulphate in non-specific gastroenteritis
Ind Med J 68: 19-23, 1974

10.)Kamat SA
Clinical trial with berberine hydrochloride for the control of diarrhea in
acute gastroenteritis
J Assoc Physicians India 15: 525-529, 1967

11.)Werbach, Melvin R and Murray, Michael T
Botanical Influences on Illness
© 1994 Third Line Press, Tarzana, California 91356

Gugulipid

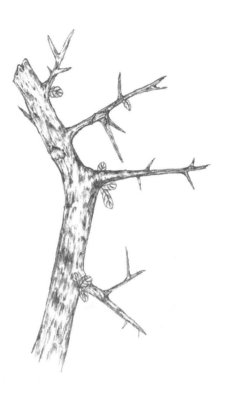

Gugulipid (*Commiphora mukul*), also known as guggul or guggulu (just gugu, no gaga) is an oleoresin from the mukul myrrh tree. It is neither a plant nor plant part; it is an exudate (sticky, liquid substance).[1] It is used extensively in Aryuvedic (Indian) medicine. Although it is from the same species, *Commiphora mukul* should not be confused with *Commiphora molmol* that is better known as myrrh, which has antiseptic properties.

Mechanism of Action:

There are two compounds, E-guggulsterone and Z-guggulsterone, which are responsible for gugulipid's cardiovascular activity. They work by increasing the liver's ability to metabolize and re-uptake LDL (low-density lipoprotein) and cholesterol from the blood stream.[2] Studies comparing gugulipid to clofibrate (Atromid-S®) have shown that serum cholesterol and triglycerides fell 11 and 17 percent, respectively, for the gugulipid and 10 and 22 percent, respectively, for the clofibrate patients. Results were seen within four to eight weeks.

Hypercholesterolemic patients responded better to gugulipid while hypertriglyceridemic patients responded better to clofibrate. One interesting note was that the HDL (the "good" cholesterol) rose in 60 percent of the patients who were taking gugulipid, while no effect was seen for the clofibrate group.[3]

Gugulipid has also been shown to have a significant lowering effect of total cholesterol and triglyceride levels, even when compared to a placebo.[3-4]

Uses:

Gugulipid has been used for the prevention and treatment of hyperlipidemia and Coronary Artery Disease (CAD). It has also been shown to be beneficial in the treatment of acne.[5]

Dosage:

A standardized extract (5 to 10 percent) should only be used in order to guarantee its potency and to avoid potential side effects. A standardized dose of 25mg three times a day with meals should be given for 12 to 16 weeks in order for benefits to be observed.

Comments:

Gugulipid is not a "magic bullet." A person should also reduce cholesterol intake by eating properly and exercising regularly— thereby keeping Coronary Artery Disease (CAD) at bay.

Gugulipid may also be used in combination with other lipid-lowering agents such as niacin (Inositol hexaniacinate works best—the "no-flush" kind), garlic, and the more powerful prescription "statins" (lovastatin, fluvastatin, and other HMG Co-A reductase inhibitors), thereby lowering their potential side-effects (muscle cramping and elevated liver enzymes). It may be beneficial to include milk thistle in this regimen in order to protect the liver. Cholesterol levels may actually *increase* when first starting to take gugulipid. This is due to the liver "dumping" its excess cholesterol into the blood stream. Don't be alarmed. This is a transient effect which will disappear the longer gugulipid is taken.

Cautions:

Minor gastrointestinal disturbances (mild diarrhea and abdominal pain) have been observed in some people. Gugulipid has also been shown to decrease platelet aggregation (stickiness) of the cells,[7] and fibrinolytic activity, so be mindful of any changes in clotting times of patients on anti-coagulant therapy.

REFERENCES: GUGULIPID

1.) Tyler, Varro E
Herbs of Choice: The Therapeutic Use of Phytomedicinals, pg. 163
© 1994 Hawthorn Press Inc., Binghamton, New York 13904-1580

2.) Nityanand S, Kapoor NK
Cholesterol lowering activity of the various fractions of Commiphora mukul (guggul)
Ind J Exp Biol 1973; 11: pg. 395-396

3.) Nityanand S et al
Clinical trials with Gugulipid; A new hypolipidemic agent
J Assoc Phys India 37(5): 323-328 1989

4.) Verma SK, Bordia A
Effects of Commiphora mukul (gum guggul) in patients of hyperlipidemia with special reference to HDL-cholesterol
Indian J Med Res 1988; 87: 356-360

5.) Dogra J et al
Oral gugulipid in acne vulgaris management
Ind J Dermatol Venereol Leprol 1990: 56 (1): 381-383

6.) Singh RB, Niaz MA, Ghosh S
Hypolipidemic and antioxidant effects of Commiphora mukul as an adjunct to dietary therapy in patients with hypercholesterolemia
Cardiovasc Drugs Ther 1994 Aug; 8 (4): 659-664

7.) Bordia A, Chuttani SK
Effect of gum guggulu on fibrinolytic activity and platelet adhesiveness in coronary artery disease
Ind Med J Res 1979; 70: 992-996

Hawthorn

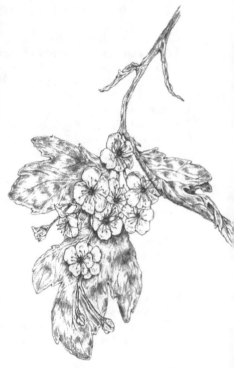

Hawthorn (*Crataegus laevigata, C. oxyacantha*) of the family Rosaceae is a shrub-like plant that is native to Europe but has now found its way to North America. The flowers are the richest source of medicinal compounds, but the leaves and berries have also been used and mixed together for synergistic effect.

Mechanism of Action:

Two main ingredients, flavonoids and oligomeric procyanidins (also known as OPCs) produce hawthorn's action. These compounds work by direct dilation of the coronary arteries and vessels. The plant does not contain any cardiac glycosides. Hawthorn has also been shown to inhibit angiotensin-converting enzyme (ACE).[1]

Uses:

Hawthorn has been shown to be effective for the following conditions:

• Decreasing resistance and improving the blood supply to the heart by dilating the coronary vessels,[2] which would be helpful in the control of angina attacks.

• Increasing exercise tolerance.[3,4]

• Increasing ejection fraction.[5] (Ejection fraction is best described as the force that the heart produces as it contracts and forces blood out from the left ventricle.)

• Improving positive inotropic effects on the heart[6] (the strength of the heart's contraction).

• Inhibiting angiotensin-converting enzyme (ACE).[1] Without this enzyme (ACE), angiotensin cannot raise the blood pressure.

• Hawthorn has also been shown to stabilize vitamin C by preventing its breakdown and therefore decrease capillary fragility.[7]

• Since one of the main side effects of ACE inhibitors is an annoying non-productive cough, hawthorn could be useful in decreasing the amount of ACE inhibitors used and thus eliminate some of the unwanted side effects.

• Hawthorn's flavonoid content has also been used to prevent the breakdown of collagen. Collagen is destroyed during the inflammatory process such as with rheumatoid arthritis, periodontal disease, and other inflammatory conditions involving bones, joints, cartilage and other connective tissues.[8] A high consumption of flavonoid compounds has been shown to be useful in reducing uric acid levels in the treatment of gout.[9] Hawthorn may hold some benefit in the treatment of this disorder.

Dosage:

A standardized extract (solid or liquid) should be used for treatment. A starting dose of 80mg twice daily can be used. Dosing may be increased upwards to 960mg a day for hard to treat cases.[10] Hawthorn may take anywhere between four to eight weeks for the effectiveness to be observed.

Comments:

Hawthorn should not be used by the patient as a "do-it-yourself" medication for cardiac problems or high-blood pressure. It should be used in conjunction with other prescribed methods of treatment (weight reduction, exercise and medication) under the supervision of a clinician. It should *not* be used during pregnancy or lactation.

Caution:

Due to hawthorn's ability to increase cardiac output, caution is advised for patients who are on beta-blockers, which decrease cardiac output.[11]

REFERENCES: HAWTHORN

1.) Uchida S, Ikari N, Ohta H, et al
   Inhibitory effects of condensed tannins on angiotensin converting   enzyme
   Jap J Pharmacol 43: 242-245, 1987

2.) Ammon HPT, Handel M
   Crataegus, Toxicology and Pharmacology
   Planta Medica 43: 101-120, 318-322, 1981

3.) Eichstadt H, Bader M, Danne O, et al
   Crataegus extract helps patients with NYHA II heart failure
   Therapiewoche 1989; 39 (45): 3288-3296

4.) Weihmayr T, Ernst E
   Therapeutic effectiveness of Crataegus
   Fortschr Med 1991 Jan 20, 114 (1-2): 27-29

5.) Weikl A, Noh H-S
   The influence of *Crataegus* on global heart failure
   Herz Gefabe 1992: 11: 516-524

6.) Popping S, Rose H, Ienescu I, Fischer Y, Kammermeier H
   Effect of a hawthorn extract on contraction and energy turnover of isolated rat cardiomyocytes
   Arzneimittelforschung 1995 Nov; 45 (11): 1157-1161

7.) Murray, Michael T
   The Healing Power of Herbs
   © 1992 Prima Publishing, Rocklin, California 95677

8.) Kuhnau J
   The flavonoids: A class of semi-essential food components: Their role in human nutrition
   Wld Rev Nutr Diet 24: 117-191, 1976

9.) Blau LW
   Cherry diet control for gout and arthritis
   Tex Rep Biol Med 8: 309-311, 1950

10.)Busse W
  Standardized Crataegus Extract Clinical Monograph
  Quart Rev Nat Med Fall 1996 pg. 189-197

11.)Schussler M, Holzl J, Fricke U
  Myocardial effects of flavonoids from Crataegus Species
  Arzneimittelforschung 1995 Aug; 45 (8): 842-845

Kava

Kava (*Peper methysticum*) also known as kava-kava, is a member of the pepper family (Piperaeae) and was given the name "intoxicating pepper" by the 18th century explorer Captain James Cook who first discovered it. It has been used for centuries in the islands of the South Pacific, especially Polynesia, Micronesia and Melanesia, as a social and ceremonial drink that was prepared from the roots of the plant. Many books and reports have been written about its use and incorporation of the herb into the customs and trade of the South Pacific. [1,2] The root and rhizome are the parts of the plant which possess its medicinal properties.

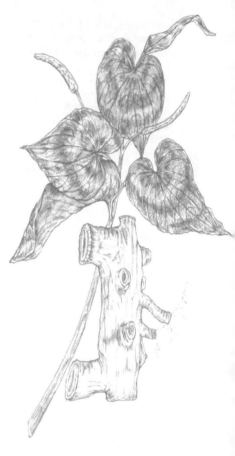

Mechanism of Action:

Kava owes its medicinal activity to a group of compounds called kavalactones or kavapyrones. Fifteen have been discovered, but six seem to be more pharmacologically active than the others. [3] This appears to be due to the fact that they are more lipophylic (fat-soluble) than the others and may account for their ability to depress spinal activity, and only affect the higher cerebral functions to a lesser degree. These compounds have been shown to reduce anxiety, promote restful sleep and relax the muscles. Other studies have shown that the kavalactones may affect the GABA-alpha receptor binding sites in different areas of the brain, possibly increasing their binding sites and their affinity for the herb.[4,5] The kavalactones have also shown some promise as an aid in the treatment of anticonvulsive disorders.[6,7]

Uses:

Kava has been used to reduce anxiety without depleting mental function as many of the benzodiazepine-type drugs (alprazolam [Xanax®], diazepam [Valium®] and chlordiazepoxide [Librium®]) do. In one study, kava was compared to oxazepam (Serax®), another benzodiazepine drug. The participants were tested for reaction time and word recognition. The group taking the kava had significantly higher scores than the group taking the oxazepam.[8] In another study, kava was compared to a placebo for the treatment of anxiety not caused by any mental disorders. The patients receiving the kava showed significant improvement even after only one week![9]

Although it has no pain-relieving properties of its own, such as the opioids, it may be helpful in skeletal muscle disorders as an adjuvant in pain management by promoting less anxiety and increased feelings of well-being and self-worth without affecting or clouding the higher mental capabilities of the brain.

Side effects:

Long term and heavy use of kava products has been shown to produce a temporary yellowing of the skin and nails and a skin rash known as kava dermopathy.[10] These side effects are all reversible once the herb is stopped or taken less frequently.

Cautions:

Pregnant or lactating women should not use kava. Because of its slight sedative effects, it should not be used in conjunction with other anti-anxiety agents, anti-depressants, anti-psychotics or alcohol. Since the skin rash that has been seen by over-indulgence of kava may be caused by an interference with cholesterol metabolism,[10] it is suggested that triglyceride and liver-function tests be performed before anyone starts taking kava.

Dosage:

A standardized extract containing 30 to 70 percent kavalactones should be taken one to two hours before bedtime to help with sleep disturbances. A standardized extract, which equals approximately 100mg, may be taken two to three times a day.

REFERENCES: KAVA

1.) Lebot V, Lindstom L, Merlin MD
Kava: The Pacific Elixir, The Definitive Guide to its Ethnobotany, History, and Chemistry
© 1997 Inner Traditions Int LTD

2.) *Kava Medicine Hunting in Paradise: The Pursuit of a Natural Alternative to Anti-Anxiety*
Drugs and Sleeping Pills
Kilham, Christopher © 1996
Inner Traditions Int LTD

3.) Smith RM, et al
"High-performance liquid chromatography of Kava lactones from *Piper Methysticum*"
Journal of Chromatography 233: 303-308, 1984

4.) Davies LP, Drew CA, Duffield P, Johnston GA, Jamieson DD
Kavapyrones and resin: studies on GABA-alpha, GABA-beta, and benzodiazepine binding sites in rodent brain
Pharmacol-Toxicol 1992 Aug; 71 (2): 120-126

5.) Jussofie-A, Schmiz-A, Hiemke
Kavapyrone enriched extract from *Piper methysticum* as modulator of GABA binding site in different regions of rat brain
Psychopharmacology-Berl 1994 Dec; 116 (4): 469-474

6.) Gleitz J, Friese J, Beile A, Ameri A, Peters T
Anticonvulsive action of (+/-)-Kavain estimated from its properties on stimulated synaptosomes and Na(+) channel receptor sites
European Journ Pharmacol 1996 Nov 7; 315 (1): 89-97

7.) Schmitz D, et al
Effects of methysticin on three different models of seizure like events studied in rat hippocampal and entorhinal cortex slices
Naunyn-Sctimiedebergs-Arch-Pharmacol 1995 April 351 (4): 348-355

8.) Munte TF, Heinze HJ, Matzke M, Steitz J
Effects of oxazepam and an extract of Kava roots (Piper Methysticum)
on related potentials in a word recognition task
Neuropsychobiology 27 (1): 46-53 1993

9.) Lehmann E, et al
"Efficacy of a special Kava extract (Piper methysticum) in patients with
states of anxiety, tension, and excitedness of non mental origin-A
double-blind Placebo-controlled Study of Four Weeks Treatment"
Phytomedicine 3 (2): 113-119

10.)Norton SA, Ruze, P
Kava dermopathy
Journal Amer Acad Dermatol 1994 July; 31 (1): 89-97

Licorice

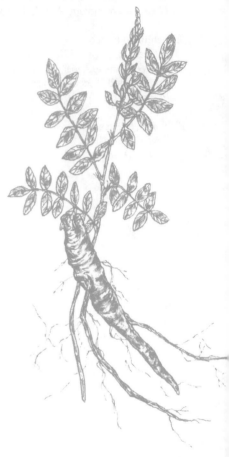

Licorice (*Glycyrrhiza glabra*) is a small shrub-like herb that grows in temperate climates.

The root holds the medicinal properties of the plant. Along with ginkgo biloba, licorice is probably the most widely used and investigated herb in all of phytotherapy. It is used alone or mixed with other herbs in combination products. It has been used for many years as a flavoring agent in the preparation of many pharmaceuticals. Unfortunately today's artificial flavoring, usually anise, is often passed off as licorice flavor.

Mechanism of Action:

Licorice contains glycyrrhizin (glycyrrhizic acid). This compound gives licorice its taste and sweetness. Licorice is actually 50 times sweeter than sugar.[1] When the body metabolizes glycyrrhizin, it is broken down to glycyrrhetic acid and two molecules of glucuronic acid.[1] Glycyrrhetic acid inhibits the enzymes that metabolize prostaglandins E^1 and F^2 alpha.[1] With an increase in these prostaglandins, peptic ulcers heal at a much faster rate.

Misoprostol (Cytotec®), a synthetic prostaglandin E^1 analog[2,5] prescription drug, has been used to prevent duodenal and gastric ulcers in patients who are on aspirin or are taking large amounts of non-steroidal anti-inflammatory drugs (NSAIDs)[3,4] such as ibuprofen or naprosyn. The problem with synthetic prostaglandins is that they increase uterine contractions and vaginal bleeding. Therefore, misoprostol should not be given to females of childbearing age unless contraceptive measures are taken.[5] This is a good indication where licorice could be used as an alternative to controlling and possibly healing the ulcer.

Uses:

The constituents in licorice display many pharmacological actions, which include:

• *Healing peptic ulcers*

Rather than inhibit the release of gastric acid as many of the histamine 2-receptor antagonists do (cimetidine, ranitidine nizatidine, and famotidine, to name a few), licorice increases the number of mucous-secreting cells (thereby increasing the amount of substances secreted) improving the quality of the mucous secreted, increasing the life span of the surface intestinal cells and enhancing the micro-circulation of the gastrointestinal tract lining.[6,7]

• *Anti-inflammatory*

Licorice has been used in the treatment of asthma, eczema and many other conditions whereby the adrenals may need help in the manufacturing of steroids.

Cautions:

Since licorice possesses aldosterone-like actions, over-use can cause sodium retention, high blood-pressure, water retention and lower potassium levels (pseudoaldosteronism).[8,9] Because of these side effects, deglycyrrhizinated licorice (DGL) should be used for therapeutic purposes. Patients should also be advised to eat a low-sodium and high-potassium diet.[10]

Glycyrrhetic acid has been shown to have a positive interaction with the hormones of the adrenal cortex. Thus, it has exhibited anti-inflammatory and anti-allergic effects similar to hydrocortisone.[11] There have also been reports of its being an adjunctive therapy in Chronic Fatigue Syndrome (CFS) and Addison's disease whereby it "jump-starts" the adrenals.[12,13]

Since licorice affects many hormonal systems, it is *not* recommended to be used during pregnancy.

Aids oral and bronchial mucous membranes

Licorice has also been shown to be an effective expectorant and exhibits very good anti-tussive properties.[14] It has also been shown that consuming oral lozenges of DGL has helped in the treatment of canker sores.[15,16] A mouth wash may also be made from the powder.

Dosage:

Deglycyrrhizinated licorice (DGL) is the safest form of licorice to use.

Gastric ulcers

Take a quarter of a teaspoonful of powder 3 to 4 times daily with meals or chew 1 to 2 tablets (250mg to 500mg) 3 times daily with meals.

Oral bronchial mucosal symptoms

Chew 1 to 2 tablets (250mg to 500mg) 3 times daily

REFERENCES: LICORICE

1.) Tyler, Varro E
   Herbs of Choice: The Therapeutic Use of Phytomedicinals, pg. 66
   © 1994 Hawthorn Press Inc, Binghamton, New York 13904-1580

2.) Young Lloyd Yee, Koda-Kimblle Mary Anne
   Applied Therapeutics-The Clinical Use of Drugs, Sixth Edition
   Applied Therapeutics Inc, Vancouver, WA
   Chpt 23 "Upper Gastrointestinal Disorders"

3.) Graham Dy, et al
Prevention of NSAID-induced gastric ulcer with misoprostol
multicentre, double-blind, placebo-controlled trial
Lancet 1988: 1277-1280

4.) Graham Dy, et al
Duodenal and gastric ulcer prevention with misoprostol in arthritis
patients taking NSAIDs
Ann Intern Med 1993; 119: 257-262

5.) Jones JB, Bailey RT
Misoprostol: a prostaglandin E analog with antisecretory and
cytoprotective properties
DICP 1989; 23: 276-282

6.) Murray , Michael T
The Healing Power of Herbs, pg. 161
© 1992 Prima Publishing, Rocklin, California 95677

7.) Reed P, Vincent-Brown A, Cook P,et al
Comparative study on carbonoxolone and cimetidine in the manage-
ment of duodenal ulcer
Acta Gastro-Enterol Belgica 46: 459-468 1983

8.) Farese RV, et al
Licorice-induced hypermineralcorticoidism
N Engl J Med 325 (17): 1223-1227 1991

9.) MacKenzie MA, et al
The influence of glycyrrhetinic acid on plasma cortisol and cortisone in
healthy young volunteers
J Clin Endocrinol Metab 70: 1637-1643, 1990

10.) Baron J, et al
Metabolic studies, aldosterone secretion rate and plasma renin after
carbenoxolone sodium as biogastrone
Br Med J 2: 793-795, 1969

11.) Mills, Simon Y.
Out of the Earth: The Essential Book of Herbal Medicine, pp. 505-510
© 1991 Penguin Books, Viking Arkana, London

12.) Brown D
Licorice Root-Potential Early Intervention for Chronic Fatigue Syndrome
NPRC Inc, Seattle, Washington 98103
Summer 1996, pp. 95-97

13.) Baschetti R
Chronic fatigue syndrome and liquorice (Letter)
New Zealand Med J 1995; 108: 156-157

14.) Chandler RF
Canadian Pharmaceutical Journal 118: 420-425 (1985)

15.) Poswillo D, Partridge M
Management of recurrent aphthous ulcers
Br Dent J 157: 55-57 1984

16.) Segal R, Pisanty S, Wormser R, Azaz E, Sela M
Anticarcinogenic activity of licorice and glycyrrhinine I: Inhibition of in vitro plaque formation by streptococcus mutans
J Pharm Sci 74: 79-81, 1985

Milk Thistle

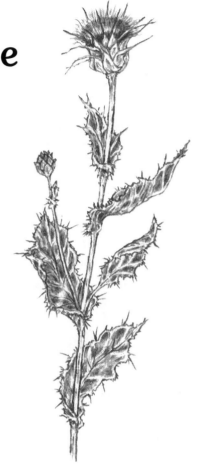

M ilk thistle *(Silybum marianum)* is native to Europe and California. It has also been called Mary thistle, Marian thistle, lady's thistle and holy thistle. Legend has it that the name *marianum* comes from the folklore that the white mottling on the leaves came from a drop of the Virgin Mary's milk.[1] The seed head of the dried flower and sometimes the leaves are used for medicinal purposes.

Mechanism of Action:

Milk thistle's active ingredient is called silymarin, which is actually a mixture of silybin, silydianin and silychristine.

Silymarin prevents liver toxic substances from penetrating into the interior of the hepatocyte (cells that make up the liver) by altering the structure of the outer cell membrane. It also enhances the regenerative ability of the liver and the formation of new hepatocytes by stimulating the action of nucleolar polymerase, resulting in an increase in ribosomal protein synthesis.[2,3]

Uses:

As mentioned previously, milk thistle (silymarin) strengthens the cell wall by binding to receptor sites on the cell. With these sites occupied by the silymarin, substances such as alcohol, [4] chemicals (carbon tetrachloride),[5] and mushroom toxins[6] cannot exert their liver-damaging effects. The effects of the deadly *Amanita phalloides* mushroom (also known as deathcap, death angel, or avenging angel) can be reversed almost 100 percent of the time even if given as long as 24 hours after ingestion! Milk thistle has been shown to have positive effects with the following conditions:

• Stimulate regeneration of liver cells damaged by alcohol or drugs. Silymarin's regenerative properties will only affect healthy cells. It will not contribute to the stimulation of cancerous cells.[7]

• Slow the advancement of liver cirrhosis.[8]

• Protection against free radical damage by increasing glutathione levels.[9]

• Guard against occupational hepatoxins.[10]

• Adjuvant therapy in the treatment of acute and chronic hepatitis.[11,12]

• Protection of the liver against hepatotoxic prescription drugs such as antidepressives and anticonvulsants.

• Protection of the liver against acetaminophen damage.[13,14]

• Protection against liver *and* kidney damage due to the chemotherapy drug cisplatin.[15,16]

Dosage:

A standardized dose of 70 to 80 percent of silymarin should be used. This equates to approximately 400 to 600mg a day in divided doses. Take with meals. Since silymarin is not very water soluble, teas should be avoided. Results are usually seen after six to eight weeks and should be verified by liver function tests. The only side effect seen with silymarin is a mild laxative effect. Because of this laxative's effect, it should not be used during pregnancy.

REFERENCES: MILK THISTLE

1.) Grieve, Mrs. M
A Modern Herbal, pg. 797
© 1931 Harcourt, Brace and Co, 1971 Dover Publication NY, NY

2.) Grauds, Constance
Milk Thistle—From: *Milk Thistle*, Constance Grauds R.Ph.
Pharmacy Times, March 1996
The Source: Fall 1996 Vol. II, No 3

3.) Wagner, H, Horhammer L, Munster R
The chemistry of silymarin (silybin), the active principle of the fruits of
Silybum marianum (L.) Gaetn
Arzneim-Forsch Drug Res 18 (1968): 688-696

4.) Ferenci P. et al
Randomized controlled trial of Silymarin treatment in patients with
cirrhosis of the liver
J Hepatology 9: 105-113, 1989

5.) Kim HJ, Chun YJ, Park JD, Kim SI, Roh JK, Jeong TC
Protection of rat liver microsomes against carbon tetrachloride-induced
lipid peroxidation by red ginseng saponin through cytochrome P 450
inhibition
Planta Med 1997 Oct; 63 (5): 415-418

6.) Carducci R, Armellin MF, Volpe C, Basile G, Caso N, Apicella A, Basile V
Silibinin and acute poisoning with *Amanita phalloides*
Minerva Anestesiol 1996 May; 62 (5): 187-193

7.) Sonnenbichler J, Goldberg M, et al
Stimulating effect of silybin on the DNA-synthesis in partially hepatecto-
mized rat livers: Non-response in hepatoma and other malignant cell lines
Biochem Pharmacol 35 (1986): 538-541

8.) DiMario FR, Farini L, et al
The effects of silymarin on the liver function parameters of patients with
alcohol-induced liver disease: a double-blind study
In: *Der Toxish-metabolische heberschaden* (de Ritis LF, Csomos G,
and Braatz R, eds), Hans. Verl-Kontor, Lubek 1981: 54-58

9.) Altorjay I, Dalmi L, Sari B, Imre S, Balla G
The effect of silibinin (Legalon) on the free radical scavenger mecha-
nisms of human erythrocytes in vitro
Acta Physiol Hung 1992; 80 (1-4): 375-380

10.) Szilard, S, Szentgyorgyi D, Demeter I
Protective effect of Legalon in workers exposed to organic solvents
Acta Med Hung 45 (2): 249-256, 1988

11.) Magliulo E, Gagliardi B, Fiori GP
Results of a double blind study on the effect of silymarin in the
treatment of acute viral hepatitis, carried out at two medical centers
Med Klin 73 (28-29): 1060-1065, 1978

12.) Mascarella S, et al
Therapeutic and antilipoperoxidant effects of silybin-phosphatidylcho
line complex in chronic liver disease: Preliminary results
Curr Ther Res 53 (1): 98-102, 1993

13.) Shear NH, Malkiewicz IM, Klein D, Koren G, Randor S, Newman MG
Acetaminophen-induced toxicity to human epidermoid cell line A431
and hepatoblastoma cell line
Hep G2, in vitro, is diminished by silymarin
Skin Pharmacol 1995; 8 (6): 279-291

14.) Muriel P, Garciapia T, Perez-Alvarez V, Mourelle M
Silymarin protects against paracetamol-induced lipid peroxidation and
liver damage
J Appl Toxicol 1992 Dec; 12 (6): 439-442

15.) Bokemeyer C, Fels LM, Dunn T, Voight W, Gaedeke J, Schmoll HJ,
Stolte H, Lentzen H
Silibinin protects against cisplatin-induced nephrotoxicity without
compromising cisplatin or ifosfamide anti-tumor activity
Br J Cancer 1996 Dec; 74 (12): 2036-2041

16.) Gaedeke J, Fels LM, Bokemeyer C, Mengs U, Stolte H, Lentzen H
Cisplatin nephrotoxicity and protection by silibinin
Nephrol Dial Transplant 1996 Jan; 11 (1): 55-62

St. John's Wort

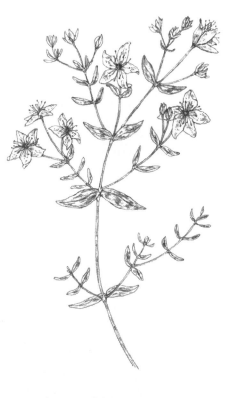

Anxiety, depression, insomnia. Someone you know is probably suffering from one on these problems. Weren't things supposed to get better as technology advanced? Well, technology has advanced but it has left a mess for us to clean up. Sometimes the mess is too overwhelming to deal with—so many people suffer from the mental and physical problems that develop when 32 hours of work and play (play?) need to be crammed into a 24-hour day.

Enter Mother Nature. Never depressed or strung out, as calm as a lake at a summer's sunset, she gives us one of her children, St. John's wort (*Hypericum perforatum, Hypericaceae*).

St. John's wort's medicinal effects have been known in Europe, especially Germany, for some time. Its success in treating mild to moderate depression with very few side effects make it a most desirable phytopharmaceutical.

Mechanism of Action:

St. John's wort acts in different ways, which may include MAO inhibitor of both types A and B,[1,2] and inhibition of the re-uptake of seratonin, noradrenaline, adrenaline and dopamine. Hypericin and pseudohypericin are the two main ingredients of a synergistic mixture that are responsible for St. John's wort's mechanism of action.

Uses:

- Mild to moderate depression[3]
- Mild to moderate anxiety
- Neuralgic pain

Studies have demonstrated that the standardized extract of St. John's wort can significantly improve symptoms of anxiety, depression, and the feelings of worthlessness. In fact, the effectiveness of the St. John's wort extract in relieving depression has been shown to be greater than that produced by standard drugs including amitriptyline and imipramine.

While these drugs (the tricyclic amines especially) are associated with significant anticholinergic side effects (most often drowsiness, dry mouth, constipation, and impaired urination), St. John's wort extract, at the usually prescribed level of intake, is not associated with these side effects. In addition to improving moods, St. John's wort has been shown to greatly enhance sleep quality.[4] St. John's wort has been combined with other products and used topically as a cream or lotion for wound healing and mild inflammation.

Dosage and Administration:

A St. John's wort extract standardized to hypericin content of 0.1 to 0.3 percent should be used. This is equivalent to approximately 300mg, one to three times daily. St. John's wort should be used for a minimum of one to two months for the benefits to be observed.

Warnings:

At higher than average dosage levels, St. John's wort may cause photosensitivity in a few individuals. Therefore it should be used with caution by fair-skinned individuals or persons who must be exposed to long periods of sunlight while carrying out their daily routine.

It's smart to take the usual precautions—wear long-sleeved clothing, use a sunblock with an SPF of at least 15, and wear a hat.

Since the mechanism of action of St. John's wort may include some MAO inhibition (although the jury's still out on this one), the following foods should be avoided:

• Tofu—especially fermented tofu, which contains high amounts of tyramine

• Aged cheese—fresh cheese, cottage and cream cheese are acceptable

• Meat extracts—contain tyramine

• Sausage, bologna, pepperoni and salami

• Sauerkraut

• Miso soup

• Brewer's yeast

• Pickled fish

• Chianti wine, vermouth, beer and ale[5,6]

Cautions:

St. John's wort should *not* be taken together with other antidepressant medications. Most prescription antidepressants have a very long half-life. In order to convert over to St. John's wort, the prescription drug should gradually be tapered down in increments of one quarter of the dose every three to four days while the St. John's wort is slowly increased to its desired dose. This should only be done under the direct supervision of a trained clinician.

REFERENCES: ST. JOHN'S WORT

1.) Hoffmann, David "Herbal Alternatives to Prozac"
Medicines from the Earth, Protocols for Botanical Healing, 1996
Official Proceedings pg. 72-76 1996

2.) Nordfors M, Hartvig P
St. John's Wort against depression in favour again
Lakartidningen 1997 June 18; 4(25): 2365-2367

3.) Linde K, Ramirez G, Mulrow CD, Pauls A, Weidenhammer W, Melchart D
St. John's Wort for depression-An overview and meta-analysis of randomized clinical trials
BMJ 1996 Aug 3; 313(7052) 253-258

4.) Werbach, Melvyn R and Murray, Michael T
Botanical influences on Illness © 1994 pg. 31

5.) Hoffmann, David "Foods to Avoid on Mao-inhibitors"
Medicines from the Earth, Protocols for Botanical Healing 1996
Official Proceedings pg. 77-79 1996

6.) Upton, Roy
American Herbal Pharmacopoeia monograph on St. John's Wort
Published in *HerbalGram*, #40, © 1997

Saw Palmetto

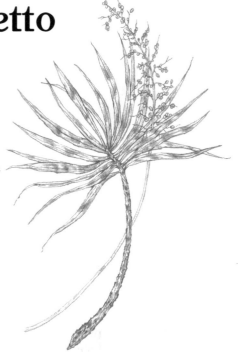

S aw palmetto, also known as *Sabal* and *Serenoa repens,* is a member of the fan palm family. It is indigenous to North America and grows predominantly along the eastern seaboard from South Carolina to Florida.[1] The plant has been used by Native Americans for genito-urinary problems. The berries are the part of the plant that is used for medicinal purposes.[2]

Mechanism of Action:

Saw palmetto inhibits the production of the enzyme 5-alpha reductase and 3-ketosteroid reductase.[3,4] These enzymes are responsible for the conversion of testosterone to the more reactive dihydrotestosterone (DHT). Saw palmetto blocks the binding of DHT to the prostate cells and thus inhibits the enlargement.

Other hormones, including estrogen may also contribute to the enlargement of the prostate. Over-consumption of meat and dairy products that have been fed estrogen during the breeding process in order to increase their weight and growth are factors affecting enlargement of the prostate. Certain pesticides that are used on fruits and vegetables may also affect the prostate. Lack of physical exercise and, according to some physicians, lack of ejaculation may also contribute to the congestion and swelling of the prostate.

Uses:

Saw Palmetto is used primarily to aid in the treatment of benign prostatic hyperplasia (BPH).[5] BPH is a non-malignant enlargement of the prostate gland and usually begins around the age of 40 through 49. It usually affects anywhere between 50 to 60 percent of the male population.[6,7] Saw palmetto may also have an anti-inflammatory effect on the prostate.

BPH is responsible for many of the following problems:

- Constricted urethra
- Dysuria
- Hesitancy
- Incomplete bladder emptying
- Nocturia
- Infections

Dosage:

A standardized extract of the liposterolic acid is recommended for the treatment of BPH. This equates to 160mg twice daily or 320mg daily with meals. Results are seen in one to two months and therapy should continue for another two to four months at which time the patient should be re-evaluated by a clinician.

Since the extract is made up of lipophilic oils, it is not recommended that a tea be used as a vehicle for the administration of the herb. Zinc (50-100mg daily) may also help shrink the prostate.[8,9] It should be taken with food to facilitate absorption.

Warnings:

Saw palmetto is *not* recommended for the treatment of bacterial prostatitis.

Side effects:

No significant side effects have been observed with the use of saw palmetto.

REFERENCES: SAW PALMETTO

1.) Murray, Michael T *The Healing Power of Herbs,* pg. 148-152
© 1992 Prima Publishing, Rocklin, California 95677

2.) Hoffmann, David L
The Herbalist, CD-ROM Version 2
© 1992 Hopkins Technology, Hopkins, MN

3.) Carilla E et al Binding of Permixon, a new treatment for prostatic benign hyperplasia, to the
cytosolic androgen receptor in the rat prostate, *J. Steroid Biochem* 20(1): 521-23, 1984

4.) Sultan, C et al Inhibition of androgen metabolism and binding by a liopsterolic extract of Serenoa repens B in human foreskin fibroblasts, *J. Steroid Biochem* 20(1):515-19, 1984

5.) Bracher, F
Phytotherapy of benign prostatic hyperplasia
Urologe A 1997 Jan:36(1):10-17

6.) Geller J, Overview of benign prostatic hypertrophy,
Urology 34, 57-68 1989

7.) Brown, Donald J *Herbal Prescriptions for Better Health*
© 1996 pg. 167-172
Prima Publishing, Rocklin, California 95677

8.) Fahim, MS et al
Zinc treatment for the reduction of hyperplasia of the prostate
Fed Proc. 35:361 1976

9.) Irving, M Bush and associates, Cook County Hospital, Chicago
Zinc and the Prostate Presented at AMA meeting, Chicago 1974

Valerian

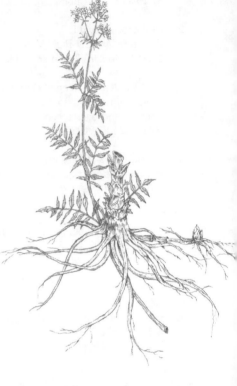

V alerian **(*Valeriana officinalis*)** is the most commonly used herb of the *valeriana* genus for its therapeutic ability. It is native to North America and Europe.

Mechanism of Action:

The plant contains constituents of volatile oils and valepotriates (valeric acid) found in the root. Studies conducted on the valeric acid have found that it weakly binds to the gamma amino benzoic acid (GABA)-alpha receptor sites in the brain and central nervous system.[1] It acts in a competitive action with any member of the family of the benzodiazepines (diazepam, alprazolam, triazolam, and chlordiazepoxide).[2] Due to valerian's weakly bound nature, it eliminates the "hang-over" effect that is usually associated with benzodiazepine usage. It has also been shown that when used for insomnia, valerian does not interfere with REM (rapid eye movement) sleep.[3]

Uses:

As adjuvant or singular therapy in the treatment of:

- Insomnia
- Anxiety
- Stress

162

- Possible withdrawal of benzodiazepine addiction (to be used only under strict clinical guidance).

Dosage and Administration:

There are many formulations of valerian, which exist at this time. Since the odor of valerian is extremely objectionable for most people, the enteric-coated tablet is recommended for better compliance. A standardized extract of at least 0.2 to 0.5 percent of valeric acid should be used.

- Insomnia: 200mg to 500mg. This should be taken approximately 1 hour before bedtime

- Anxiety and stress: 200mg to 300mg twice a day

Many valerian products are usually combined with other relaxants such as chamomile, hops, lemon balm (*Melissa officinalis*) and passion flower (*Passiflora incarnata*).[4]

Warnings:

Although valerian has been shown not to interfere with the ability to drive or to do tasks that require agility, it would be advisable not to drive or consume alcohol while taking valerian preparations.[5]

Contraindications:

Do not mix with benzodiazepine derivatives otherwise no other contraindications have been noted.

Pregnancy:

Valerian has been used during pregnancy and lactation.

REFERENCES: VALERIAN

1.) Mennini T, Bernasconi P, et al
"In vitro study on the interaction of extracts and pure compounds from *Valeriana officinalis* roots with GABA, benzodiazepine and barbiturate receptors
Fitoterapia 64: 291-300, 1993

2.) Holzl J and Godau P
Receptor binding studies with *Valeriana officinalis* on the benzodiaz

epine receptor
Planta Med 55: 642, 1989

3.) Leathwood PD, et al
Aqueous extract of Valerian root (*Valeriana officinalis L.*) improves sleep quality in man
Pharmacol Biochem Behavior 17 (1): 65-71, 1982

4.) Dressing H, Riemann D, et al
Insomnia: Are Valerian/Melissa combinations of equal value to benzodiazepine?
Therapiewoche 42 PP 726-736 © 1992

5.) Gerhard U, Linnenbrink N, Georghiadou C, Hobi V
Vigilance-decreasing effects of 2 plant-derived sedatives
Schweiz Rundsch Med Prax April 9; 85 (15): 473-481, 1996

PART THREE

TOPICAL
HERBAL
TREATMENTS

TOPICAL HERBAL TREATMENTS

External preparations in the form of creams, oils and ointments have been a mainstay in herbal therapy. Many herbs that would produce serious side effects if taken internally, can usually be applied externally without serious consequences. These herbs can be found singularly or in combination with other healing herbs such as echinacea or St. John's wort.

Aloe Vera

Aloe (*Aloe barbadensis*) has been used for centuries in the treatment of many skin conditions. It was even mentioned in the New Testament of the Bible as a mixture of "myrrh and aloes" and was used to anoint Jesus' body before it was put into the tomb.[1] Aloe owes its medicinal effects to over 200 compounds but especially to its polysaccharide components especially acemannan.

There are many products on the market, which contain aloe in some way, shape or form, but nothing beats the pure product. (If you want a rough idea as to how much aloe, or any other ingredient is in a product, just look to see where it falls in the list of ingredients. If it is near the top, then it is usually a major component of the product, if it is near the bottom, then it probably contains very little.) Aloe has shown promise in helping to heal psoriasis,[2] burns, frostbite,[3] and leg ulcers.[4]

166

Caution:

One study has shown that aloe should not be used for deep puncture wounds and vertical surgical wounds such as those produced by Cesarean delivery. It actually delayed the healing process.[5] Calendula may be a better choice in these circumstances.

REFERENCES: ALOE VERA

1.) Gospel According to John 19 verses 38-42
Good News Bible
© 1976 American Bible Society

2.) Syed TA, Ahmad SA, Holt AH, et al
Management of psoriasis with *aloe vera* extract in a hydrophilic cream: a placebo-controlled, double-blind study
Tropical Med International Health 1996; 1: 505-509

3.) Heggers JP, Pelley RP, Robson MC
Beneficial effects of Aloe in wound healing
Phytother Res 7: 548-552, 1993

4.) Klein AD, Penneys NS
Aloe Vera
J Amer Acad Dermatol 18: 714-719, 1988

5.) Schmidt JM, Greenspoon JS
"Aloe vera dermal wound gel is associated with a delay in wound healing"
Ostet Gynecol 78: 115-117, 1991

6.) Roberts DB, Travis EL
Acemannan-containing wound dressing gel reduces radiation-induced skin reactions in C3H mice
Int J Radiat Oncol Biol Phys © 1995 July 15; 32 (4): 1047-1052

Apple Cider Vinegar

I won't go into great detail about some of the ailments reported to be helped by apple cider vinegar. (I've noted some references in the bibliography, reference 1,2). It has been used for everything from an astringent for skin problems, to a conditioner for the hair and scalp, and even to help in the condition of achlorhydria (a condition of decreased hydrochloric acid in the stomach leading to poor digestion and absorption of vital nutrients from our food).

I usually suggest mixing one ounce of apple-cider vinegar with 15 ounces of non-chlorinated water and using this for skin problems. Do not put this on any open wounds because it will sting. Make sure that you obtain "pure" apple cider vinegar. You can usually tell the difference because, like a good "apple cider," it is very cloudy. Don't buy the clear one since all of the beneficial ingredients have been filtered out.[2-4]

REFERENCES: APPLE CIDER VINEGAR

1.) Mindell Earl L, John Larry M
   Amazing Apple Cider Vinegar: The Medicinal Miracle, Plus the
   Curative, Cleaning and Cooking Virtues of Vinegars from Around the
   World
   Keats Publishing © 1997

2.) Bragg Paul C, Bragg Patricia
   The Miracles of Apple Cider Vinegar Health System
   Health Science Publications © 1992

Arnica

Arnica (*Arnica montana*), also known as leopard or wolf's bane, is an excellent topical agent that can be used to help decrease inflammation that is produced by sprains and bruises caused by trauma. It contains sesquiterpene lactones[1] and polysaccharides,[2,3] that are responsible for its actions. The oil is extracted from the flowers and roots. It stimulates the peripheral circulation of the blood. Arnica can be used as a cream alone or it sometimes can be mixed with other topical herbs such as calendula or witch hazel. It is also available as pure oil. The only form of arnica that can be taken internally is the homeopathic preparations. The pure plant can display toxic effects on the gastro-intestinal tract and central nervous system.

REFERENCES: ARNICA

1.) Puhlman J, Wagner H
   Immunologically Active Polysaccharides from Arnica Montana Herbes
   and Tissue Cultures
   Planta Medica 1989; 55:99

2.) *Merfort I*
   1,4,5-Tricaffeoylquinic Acid and New Flavonoid Glycosides from Arnicae
   Flos DAB9
   Planta Medica 1989;55:608

3.) Duke JA
   Handbook of Medicinal Herbs
   Boca Raton, Fl; CRC Press, 1985

Calendula

Calendula officinalis is better known as marigold. The Latin name was derived by the ancient Romans because these flowers bloomed on the day of the full moon called "calends" which was the first day of the month on the Roman calendar.[1,2]

The flowers are used medicinally. Calendula can be used for all minor skin irritations and problems and in wound healing.[3] It has mild anti-fungal, anti-inflammatory and anti-bacterial properties.

Calendula has also been used to help heal fresh scars from surgery. This has shown especially promising results. It has been recommended as a treatment for scarring caused by episiotomy or Cesarean section.[4-6] It is also used for hemorrhoids. The tincture can be mixed with a little water and used as a mouthwash to treat infections of the mouth and gums.[7]

REFERENCES: CALENDULA

1.) Grieve, Mrs M
   A Modern Herbal , pg. 517
   © 1931 Harcourt, Brace and Co, 1971 Dover Publication, NY, NY

2.) Antol, Marie Nadine
   The "T" Factor
   Energy Time Vol 7, No 3, 3/97

3.) Patrick KFM, Kumar S, Edwardson PAD, Hutchinson JJ
   "Induction of vascularisation by an aqueous extract of the flowers of *Calendulla officinalis*"
   Phytomed 1996; 3: 11-18

4.) Moskowitz R
   "Homeopathic Medicines for Pregnancy and Childbirth"
   Berkeley: North Atlantic, 1992

5.) Castro M
   "Homeopathy for Pregnancy, Birth, and the First Year"
   New York: St. Martins, 1993

6.) Ullman MPH, Dana
   "Pregnant and Laboring Women"
   Quarterly Review of Natural Medicine, Fall, 1995 pp 235-239

7.) Mills, Simon Y.
   Out of the Earth: The Essential Book of Herbal Medicine
   © 1991 Penguin Books, Viking Arkana, London

Capsicum (Capsaicin)

When you mention to someone that the use of "hot peppers" applied externally may help with the pain of arthritis, the usual response is "Do I have to eat them too?" The word capsicum is derived from the Greek "to bite" which pretty much describes its properties.[1] Capsaicin, the active ingredient, works by lessening the amount of the neurotransmitter substance P. Substance P carries the transmission of pain along the peripheral nerves to the spinal column and therefore gives us the perception of pain.

Capsaicin has been used for arthritic pain,[2] although one study has shown that capsaicin was more effective in osteoarthritis than rheumatoid arthritis.[3] It has also been used for back aches, sprains, strains, pain associated with shingles (*Herpes zoster*),[4,5] diabetic neuropathy, especially in the feet, post-mastectomy pain,[6] psoriasis,[7] and cluster headaches.[8] In order to get the full benefit of capsaicin, it should be applied at least four to five times a day until pain relief is achieved. This could take three to four weeks, so be patient. After relief is noticed, it can be applied less often. It is strongly recommended that the ointment be applied with gloves and that eye and facial contact be avoided.

REFERENCES: CAPSAICIN

1.) Grieve, Mrs M
   A Modern Herbal
   © 1931 Harcourt, Brace and Co, 1971 Dover Publication, NY, NY

2.) Deal CL, et al
   Treatment of arthritis with topical capsaicin: a double blind trial
   Clin Ther 13 (3): 383-395

3.) McCarthy GM, McCarty DJ
   "Effect of topical capsaicin in the therapy of painful osteoarthritis of the hands"
   J Rheumatol 19 (4): 604-607, 1992

4.) Bernstein JE, Korman NJ, Bickers DR, Dahl MV, Millikan LE
"Topical capsaicin treatment of chronic post-herpetic neuralgia"
J Amer Acc Dermatology 1989 pp. 265-270

5.) Don PC
"Topical capsaicin for the treatment of neuralgia associated with herpes zoster infection"
J Amer Acc Dermatology, May 1988 pp. 1135-1136

6.) Watson CP, Evans RJ
"The post-mastectomy pain syndrome and topical capsaicin: a randomized trial"
Pain 51 (3): 375-379, 1992

7.) Ellis CN, Berberian B, et al
A double-blind evaluation of topical capsaicin in pruritic psoriasis
J Amer Acad Dermatol 29: 438-442 1993

8.) Marks DR, et al
"A double-blind placebo-controlled trial of intranasal capsaicin for cluster headache."
Cephalalgia 13 (2): 114-116 1993

Lavender

Most people have come in contact with the fragrant odor of lavender (*Lavandula angostifolia*) in some way, shape, or form. It has been a mainstay in the cosmetics industry for decades. Pure lavender oil can be used externally and aromatically as a calming agent on the central nervous system. A drop or two of pure oil rubbed into the temples may help relieve a headache by relaxing the body and relieving the tension. It may also be used in the bath to promote a relaxing effect. The oil should only be used **Externally**. If it is too strong, two drops of oil can be mixed with 5 ml (1 teaspoonful) of carrier oil such as almond or vegetable oil (*don't* use petroleum-based oils—they actually dry out and may irritate the skin).

Tea Tree Oil

*M*elaleuca alternifolia, also known as Australian tea tree, and Ti tree, is a small shrub native to only one place on the planet—New South Wales, Australia.[1] Because of its antiseptic properties, tea tree oil was even included in the first aid kits of British and Australian soldiers during World War II.[2] Another specific use of the oil is as an effective anti-fungal. A study was conducted comparing tea tree oil with Tolnaftate, a product commonly used for the treatment of athletes' foot (*tinea pedis*) and a placebo. The Tolnaftate and tea tree oil groups showed significant improvement over the placebo group.[3]

Another study was conducted comparing the oil with 5 percent benzoyl peroxide in the treatment of acne. Both groups showed significant improvement especially the tea tree group, which reported less irritating effects (burning, itching, skin irritation) than the benzoyl peroxide group.[4]

Other uses of tea tree oil include:

- Cold sores—swab lesions 3 to 4 times daily
- Insect repellent
- Insect bites—swab oil on the bite
- Nail infections—soak fingers in oil and dab area 2 to 3 times daily

There have been some concerns recently with respect to the quality of tea tree oil. Many products have been adulterated with other oils with no medicinal value. When purchasing the oil, make sure that it has been standardized by either the American Tea Tree Oil Association or by the Australian Association and that it contains 100 percent pure oil. With this percentage, you can dilute it, which is recommended, to any strength you wish with pure olive oil or other suitable vegetable oil. (Don't use petroleum-based oils like mineral oil. It actually makes the skin drier).

Quality oil should be clear with a slight yellow hue. Like any oil, it should be kept in a dark container in order to prevent it from becoming rancid. There have been some reports of people developing skin sensitivity to the oil. This will usually subside after the oil is discontinued.

REFERENCES: TEA TREE OIL

1.) Murray, Michael T
   The Healing Power of Herbs pp. 218-220
   © 1992 Prima Publishing, Rocklin, California 95677

2.) "Nature's Ultimate Antiseptic: Tea Tree Oil"
   Energy Times Vol 17 No 2 © 1997

3.) Tong MM, Altman PM and Barnetson RS
   "Tea tree oil in the treatment of tinea pedis"
   Austral J Derm 33: 145-149, 1992

4.) Bassett, IB, et al
   A comparative study of tea tree oil versus benzoyl peroxide in the treatment of acne
   Med J Aust 153: 455-458, 1990

Witch Hazel

Witch hazel *(Hamamelis virginiana)* is a Native American tree. The solution is prepared by steam distillation of the leaves and twigs. Unfortunately, the process of distilling the plant removes most of the tannins, which give the solution its healing properties. In most cases, "distilled" Witch hazel's properties are usually attributed to its high alcohol content and not from its natural ingredients. If you can find it, buy "undistilled" or "unrefined" witch hazel.[1] It is an excellent astringent for scrapes and local skin inflammations such as sunburn.

I usually suggest that patients keep a small child-resistant bottle (appropriately labeled and with the cautionary statement **"For**

External Use Only" in big letters) in the refrigerator. In this manner, the cold application adds to the healing properties of the solution, especially in decreasing the swelling from insect bites[1] and hemorrhoids. It may be applied three to four times daily.

REFERENCES: WITCH HAZEL

1.) Tyler, Varro E
Herbs of Choice: The Therapeutic Use of Phytomedicinals, pp. 151-152
© 1994 Hawthorn Press Inc, Binghamton, New York 13904-1580

APPENDIX A

EQUATIONS TO CALCULATE CHILDREN'S DOSAGES

Clark's Rule:

$$\frac{\text{Weight (lb.)}}{150} \times \text{adult dose} = \text{child's dose}$$

Young's Rule: (for children 2 years and older):

$$\frac{\text{Age(in years)}}{\text{Age (in years)} + 12} \times \text{adult dose} = \text{child's dose}$$

Body Surface Area:

$$\frac{\text{Body surface Area of child}}{1.73} \times \text{adult dose} = \text{child's dose}$$

(1.73 meter sq. = average body surface area of an adult)

Caution:
Children are not adults who wear smaller sizes! Always consult with a trained clinician before administering any medicinal herbs to children.

APPENDIX B

HERBS THAT MAY CAUSE A LAXATIVE EFFECT

- Balmony
- Barberry
- Bilberry
- Boneset
- Cascara Sagrada
- Damiana
- Dandelion root
- Elder
- Figwort
- Goldenseal
- Milk Thistle
- Oregon Grape
- Psyllium
- Rhubarb Root
- Senna
- Yellow Dock

All of these herbs may also affect a child if he or she is being breast-fed.

APPENDIX C

HERBS THAT MAY AFFECT CLOTTING TIMES

Herbs which increase clotting time:

- Astragalus
- Bilberry
- Bromelain
- Capsaicin
- Chestnut leaf
- Curcumin (tumeric)
- Evening Primrose Oil
- Feverfew
- Ginger
- Ginkgo Biloba
- Gugulipid
- Horse Chestnut
- Quercetin
- Sassafras
- Scullcap
- Sheep Sorrel

Herbs which decrease clotting time:

- Cinnamon
- Parsley

Herb which can increase *or* decrease clotting time:

- Ginseng

All of the above herbs should be held suspect if there is any change in clotting time while taking anti-coagulation therapy (Warfarin, Coumadin®). These herbs are sometimes found in combination with other herbs in order to increase their medicinal effects.[1-3]

REFERENCES: HERBS AFFECTING CLOTTING

1.) Agricultural Research Service
    Phytochemical and Ethnobotanical Databases USDA-ARS-NGRL
    Stephen M Beckstrom-Sternberg and James A Duke
    www.ars-grin.gov/~ngrlsb/index.html

2.) *Mills, Simon Y*
Out of the Earth: The Essential Book of Herbal Medicine
© 1991 Penguin Books, Viking Arkana, London

3.) Janetzky K, Morreale A P
Probable interaction between warfarin and ginseng
Am J Health-Sys Pharm Vol. 54 Mar 15 1997 pg. 692-693

APPENDIX D

HERBS AND PREGNANCY

Sound medical practice would dictate that medication be given to a pregnant patient *only* if absolutely necessary. Some people may feel that since herbs are plants they may pose less of a threat to the developing fetus. This absurd notion could not be further from the truth! People don't seem to think of tobacco as a plant but look at all the damage it does. The following is a partial list of herbs that should **never be used when pregnant.** Be especially careful with combining products.[1,2]

- Aloe (internally)
- Barberry
- Black cohosh
- Blue cohosh
- Cascara sagrada
- Dong Quai
- Ephedra (Ma Huang)
- Feverfew
- Ginkgo biloba (EGb)
- Ginseng (all forms)
- Goldenseal
- Hawthorn

- Kava
- Licorice
- Milk thistle
- Oregon Grape
- Parsley (OK as a flavoring agent)
- Pennyroyal
- Psyllium seeds (Plantago)
- Red clover
- Rue
- Senna
- Tansy
- Uva Ursi (bearberry)

REFERENCES: HERBS AND PREGNANCY

1.) Mills, Simon Y.
Out of the Earth: The Essential Book of Herbal Medicine
© 1991 Penguin Books, Viking Arkana, London

2.) Weed, Susan S.
Wise Woman for the Childbearing Years
© 1986 Ash Tree Publishing, Woodstock, NY

APPENDIX E

SURFING THE NET

If you have access to the World Wide Web of the Internet, you can find hundreds of web sites on herbal and medicinal therapy. Since web sites sprout up and disappear faster than dandelions, it would not be advantageous to list them here.

The best way to find out information is to use a search engine (Lycos, Excite, Magellan, Hot Bot, etc.) and type in the name of the herb. For example, you can use either the common name (dandelion) or its botanical name (*Taraxacum officinale*). You will find everything from the medicinal use, to growing herbs, how to use them in cooking, to selling and buying them. There are also some news groups under "alt." (for "alternate") that may also be of help.

If you are looking for specific medical information, then your best bet would be to search the Medline database. This can be accessed through Medical Matrix at <www.medmatrix.org/index.stm> or through the National Library of Medicine at <www.nlm.nih.gov>.

APPENDIX F

RECOMMENDED READING: BOOKS

Werbach, Melvin R., Murray Michael T.
Botanical Influences on Illness
© 1994 Third Line Press, Tarzana, California 91356

Murray, Michael
The Healing Power of Herbs
© 1992 Prima Publishing, Rocklin, California 91356

Brown, Donald J.
Herbal Prescriptions for Better Health
© 1996 Prima Publishing, Rocklin, California 95677

Tyler, Varro E.
Herbs of Choice: The Therapeutic Use of Phytomedicinals
© 1994 Hawthorn Press Inc., Binghamton, New York 13904

Tierra, Lesley
The Herbs of Life: Health and Healing using Western and Eastern Techniques
© 1992 The Crossing Press, Freedom, CA 95019

Grieve, Mrs. M.
A Modern Herbal
© 1931 Harcourt, Brace and Co., 1971 Dover Publication, NY, NY.

Werbach, Melvin R.
Nutritional Influences on Illness
© 1996 Second Edition, Third Line Press, Tarzana, California

Mills, Simon Y.
Out of the Earth: The Essential Book of Herbal Medicine
© 1991 Penguin Books, Viking Arkana, London

Balch, James F., Balch, Phyllis A.
Prescription for Nutritional Healing
© 1990 Avery Publishing Group, Garden City Park, NJ

PERIODICALS

HerbalGram The Journal of the American Botanical Council and the Herb Research Foundation
PO Box 144345
Austin, TX 78714-4345
(512) 926-2345
<www.herbalgram.org>

Phytomedicine International Journal of Phytotherapy and Phytopharmacology
VHC Publishers, Inc.
303 N.W. 12th Ave.
Deerfield Beach, FL 33442-1705

Medical Herbalism A Clinical Newsletter for Clinical Practitioners
PO Box 33080
Portland, OR 97233

Planta Medica
Natural Products and Medicinal Plant Research
381 Park Ave. South
NY, NY 10016

The Protocol Journal of Botanical Medicine
PO Box 108
Harvard, MA 01451
800-466-5422

Quarterly Review of Natural Medicine
Natural Product Research Consultants, Inc.
600 First Ave. Suite 205
Seattle, WA 98104

The Review of Natural Products
Facts and Comparisons
111 West Port Plaza, Suite 300
St. Louis, MO 63146-3098
800-223-0553

The Source A Newsletter of the Association of Natural Medicine Pharmacists
Association of Natural Medicine Pharmacists
PO Box 150727
San Rafael, CA 94915-0727
(415) 453-3534

APPENDIX G

ORGANIZATIONS

American Association of Naturopathic Physicians
2366 Eastlake Ave. East, Suite 322
Seattle, WA 98102
(206) 323-7610

American Botanical Council   <www.herbalgram.org>
PO Box 144345
Austin, TX 78714-4345
(512) 926-2345

American Herb Association
PO Box 1673
Nevada City, CA 95959

American Herbalists Guild
Box 1683
Soquel, CA 95073
(408) 464-2441

American Holistic Medical Association
4101 Lake Boone Trail # 201
Raleigh, NC 26707
(919) 787-5146

Association of Natural Medicine Pharmacists
PO Box 150727
San Rafael, CA 94915-0727
(415) 453-3534
<www.anmp.org>

Herbal Research Foundation
1007 Pearl Street, Suite 200
Boulder, CO 80302
(303) 449-2265

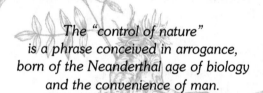

*The "control of nature"
is a phrase conceived in arrogance,
born of the Neanderthal age of biology
and the convenience of man.*

—Rachel Carson (1907-1964)
from *The Silent Spring*

Index

A

Acidophilus 133
ACE inhibitors 100, 139
Acne 29, 136
Acupuncture 33
Addison's disease 148
Allergies 29
Allicin 112
Alliin 112
Alliinase 112
Aloe vera 60, 166
Alzheimer's disease 120, 121
Antioxidants 90, 120
Anxiety 30, 95, 142, 155-6, 162
Apigenin 96
Apple cider vinegar 168
Arnica 169
Arthritis 31
Aspergillus 112
Asthma 32, 120, 147
  and breathing exercises 33
  and diet and exercise 33
  and relaxation techniques 33
Astragalus 33, 59, 87
Atherosclerosis 34, 122
  and angina 34
  and diet and exercise 34
  and heart attack 34
  and high-blood pressure 34

B

Bacillus cereus 112
Benign breast pain 52

Benign prostatic hyperplasia (BPH)
  34, 160
Berberis 82
Bilberry 37, 43-4, 68-9, 90
Bioflavonoids 90
Black cohosh 48, 64
  and gynecological disorders 48
Bromelain 31
Burns 166

C

Calcium 64
Calendula 55, 60, 169
Candida albicans 103, 112
Candidiasis 35
Canker sores 36
Capsaicin 31, 72, 171
Cardiovascular issues 112, 139
Cascara sagrada 40
Cataracts 36, 68, 91
Celery 82
Cerebral insufficiencies 121
Cerebrovascular disorders 37
Chamomile 30, 36, 46, 61, 94
Chemotherapy 88, 117, 152
Children's dosages 176
Chronic fatigue syndrome 103,
  128, 148
Circulatory problems 120
Clotting times 178
Colds 88, 103
Colic 95

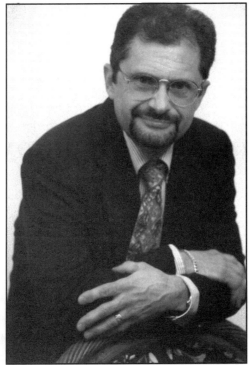

Linda Chestney

Steven Ottariano, R.Ph.

About the Author

As a practicing clinical pharmacist, Steve Ottariano understands the benefits of combining traditional "Western" pharmacy with the age-old wisdom of medicinal plants. The synergy of the two disciplines is often more effective than either one in isolation. His traditional scientific training, along with years of in-depth study of medicinal herbal therapies, means Ottariano is well qualified to integrate the valuable knowledge he brings in his book. Ottariano offers the reader not only substantiated scientific studies, but also his own personal experiences.

An accomplished lecturer, he has helped thousands of people and shown them the benefits herbal therapy offers. He also lectures frequently at New England-area hospitals and colleges, including Massachusetts College of Pharmacy. Additionally, his unique perspective and wealth of information is frequently sought out by the media as an expert source.

Ottariano is a certified martial arts instructor holding black belts in two traditional styles of Karate (Shorin-ryu and Goju-ryu) and is a member of the Association of Natural Medicine Pharmacists.

191

Want another copy?

If you'd like to purchase a copy of this book, please check with your local book store or write to the address below. A FREE catalog of Nicolin Fields Publishing, Inc.'s books is also available—just drop us a note.

To order this book directly from the publisher, send a check, money order or your credit card number and expiration date for $14.95 plus $3.50 for postage for one book ($1.00 for each additional book). Please allow two weeks for delivery.

Nicolin Fields Publishing, Inc.
2456 Lafayette Road
Portsmouth, NH 03801

603 422-8772
outside of New Hampshire,
call 800 333-9883 (orders only)
nfp@nh.ultranet.com

Please also note that the author is available as an expert resource for media interviews. Please call the publisher if you would like to arrange an interview.